REACTIONS TO MOTHERHOOD
The role of post-natal care

'For this reason I kneel before the Father, from whom the whole family in heaven and on earth derives its name. I pray that out of his glorious riches he may strengthen you with power through his Spirit and your inner being.'
Ephesians 3:14–16

Reactions to motherhood

THE ROLE OF POST-NATAL CARE

JEAN A. BALL

Director of Research, North Lincolnshire Health Authority

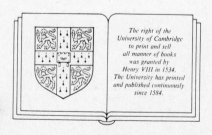

The right of the
University of Cambridge
to print and sell
all manner of books
was granted by
Henry VIII in 1534.
The University has printed
and published continuously
since 1584.

CAMBRIDGE UNIVERSITY PRESS

Cambridge

London   New York   New Rochelle

Melbourne   Sidney

Published by the Press Syndicate of the University of Cambridge
The Pitt Building, Trumpington Street, Cambridge CB2 1RP
32 East 57th Street, New York, NY 10022, USA
10 Stamford Road, Oakleigh, Melbourne 3166, Australia

First published 1987

Printed in Great Britain by Redwood Burn Ltd., Trowbridge, Wiltshire.

British Library cataloguing in publication data
Ball, Jean A.
Reactions to motherhood: the role of post-natal care
1. Postnatal care   2. Midwives
I. Title
618.6   RG950

Library of Congress cataloguing in publication data
Ball, Jean A.
Reactions to motherhood.
Bibliography: p.
Includes index.
1. Postnatal care – Psychological aspects.
2. Motherhood – Psychological aspects.   3. Midwives.
I. Title   [DNLM: 1. Midwifery.   2. Mothers – psychology
3. Postnatal Care.   WQ 500 B187r]
RG801.B234   1987   155.6'463   86–17165

ISBN 0 521 30331 1 hard covers
ISBN 0 521 31629 4 paperback

MU

Contents

Foreword

I am pleased and honoured to be asked to write this introduction for Jean Ball's long-awaited book. I have known and admired Jean Ball for many years as we have both been working in the East Midlands, involved in the training of midwives and doctors. We share a conviction that a woman's experience of childbirth, pregnancy and the immediate puerperium plays a pivotal and essential part in her adjustment to motherhood and her enjoyment of her new child; it is also probably an important risk factor for those who are vulnerable to post-natal mental illness. We both belong to the Marce Society, an international scientific society founded in 1980 to promote the understanding, prevention and treatment of mental illness related to childbearing. Hundreds of professionals, psychiatrists, obstetricians, psychologists, social workers and midwives, now belong to this society; many of its members are actively engaged in research which ultimately will lead to the more effective detection and prevention of post-natal mental illness, its more effective treatment, and ways of enhancing the emotional well-being of the mother and child.

The results of Jean Ball's research are already well known to many people. They carry conviction not only because of the methodology but also because of their face validity. She puts forward her views in meetings and lectures with practical good humour and an earthy common sense, and her results and ideas have significantly altered midwifery practice, certainly locally in the East Midlands.

Mental illness after childbirth is common. Many reputable recent research studies suggest that an incidence of at least 16% is standard, not only in Britain but also in many other countries. Sixteen per cent of all recently delivered women suffer from a severity of emotional distress and disturbance of functioning for a sufficiently lengthy period of time to rate as a 'case' of psychiatric illness. This figure does not include the countless thousands of women who are less disturbed but who are none-the-less miserable and do not enjoy their baby or their life as a mother as they should. One-third of the women who suffer from mental illness after childbirth would benefit from treatment but the majority is not treated and only a relatively small proportion is admitted to a hospital. Although many of the factors that we know to be associated with the most severe forms of mental illness are outside both the patient's and the caretaker's control, we do know many things about both the severe and the milder forms of illness which allow us to predict at least a vulnerable group of women. We should be able to offer these women extra support and perhaps even to intervene and reduce the risk of their becoming mentally ill. At the very least we should be able to detect their illness at an early stage and treat it promptly and effectively. In her book, Jean Ball identifies some of the risk factors ante-natally and I hope that people who read this book will be better able to detect the highly anxious woman and to help her reduce her levels of anxiety before delivery. Common sense as well as clinical experience tells us that profound disappointment in the process of childbirth increases the risk of women becoming post-natally depressed and that conversely a pleasurable and positive experience of childbirth should reduce this risk.

The fascinating studies of Marshall Klaus that Jean Ball refers to throughout her book have shown us that in many different cultures, the continuous presence of a warm, supportive person throughout delivery, who is able to love and help the delivering woman and encourage her during the phase of delivery, significantly reduces the length of time spent in labour and the need for surgical intervention. The fact that so many of these ladies, called by Marshall Klaus '*doulas*', become godparents after delivery is a testimony to the relationships that were cemented during labour. It would be logical to assume that such social support during labour would also improve maternal well-being and enjoyment of the child after delivery. Many of us who have watched Professor Klaus's films and listened to his lectures have been struck by the similarities between the behaviour of his *doulas* and the ideal behaviour of a British midwife.

Jean Ball comments in her book on the sense of gratitude that patients feel for the continuous presence of a midwife throughout labour. If our midwives could be encouraged to add to their technical competence the capacity to act as a *doula*, then I am sure they would have a significant effect on the mental health of mothers after delivery.

All professionals involved in the care of the pregnant delivering woman, be they doctors or midwives, must have sound working knowledge of the emotional needs and changes of the pregnant woman. This is as essential for her well-being as their knowledge of her physical needs. Now that the tragedy of maternal and infant death is a rarity, all of our patients have a right not only to a safe delivery and a healthy infant, but also to an experience that is as positive as possible, is regarded by everybody as being dignified and precious, and is conducted by a loving and familiar person who is technically competent and aware of their needs. These people should have the skills and resources to recognise the validity of emotional needs during this most important period of transition in a lifetime and be able to deal with them effectively.

I hope that this book will be read by every student midwife and every doctor who is training for either the speciality of obstetrics or primary health care, but in particular I hope that it will be read by those consultant obstetricians and senior nurses who are responsible for the organisation of maternity services.

Margaret Oates
Senior Lecturer and Consultant
University of Nottingham Medical School

Preface

This book arose from a desire to learn more about the emotional needs of women as they take on the demanding role of motherhood. My training as a midwife had not given me any information about the psychological processes which underlie transition to motherhood; indeed most midwifery and obstetric textbooks lead one to assume that once the baby is safely born, the mother is instantly able to cope with her new role. The textbooks discuss the physiological processes of the puerperium, the nutritional needs of the infant and something of the formation of maternal–child relationships, but virtually nothing about how to help a woman cope with the varying demands and expectations which mothering brings.

A perusal of research about post-natal depression gave me some insight into emotional processes, and the importance of peer and family support, but there was very little about the care and support which midwives give during the post-natal period, and the effect which this might have upon transition to motherhood. This is surprising when one considers that midwives support mothers through the childbearing process in all societies and have done since the beginning of recorded history!

The research which followed and which forms the basis of this book was designed to bridge those gaps; to learn more about the effects which psychological and social factors and the care given by midwives might have upon emotional needs of mothers during the first six weeks of their infants' lives; and to help midwives and other care-givers to make the emotional support of women an integral part of the care they give. The research traced the experiences of 279 women from the thirty-sixth week of pregnancy until six weeks after the birth of the baby, and included the perceptions which mothers and midwives had about each other and about the transition to motherhood. The book does not enter into the arguments about the merits of home versus hospital delivery, but concentrates its attention upon those who, like the majority of women in this country, give birth in hospital and then receive post-natal care via the hospital and community midwifery services.

Many different factors influence a woman's reactions to motherhood, and in order to understand the interaction of such factors and to evaluate the role played by post-natal care it was necessary to apply a strict discipline of statistical analysis to what is a fundamentally subjective process. By this means I hoped to place the midwifery aspects of the study within the context of previous studies of the emotional reaction to motherhood, and to avoid interpreting the results in line with my own feelings and cherished beliefs. There is also need for midwives to be more objective in their evaluation of their role and practice. The book contains, therefore, as much statistical evidence for its assertions as will satisfy the demands of a scientific approach to the subject, but not so much as to obscure the essence of the deeply personal experience of motherhood. I hope that those who are irritated by statistics will forgive their inclusion and perhaps appreciate their ability to illumine and add weight to argument and discussion, and that those who rely greatly upon them will appreciate that there are many things which cannot be measured.

This book would not have been written without the help of many people, to whom I wish to express my thanks. Firstly, I would like to thank the 279 mothers who shared their experiences with me, and the midwives and obstetricians who allowed me to observe their work; the Department of Health and Social Security who funded the research, and Margorie and George Amans.

My thanks also go to those who supervised the research: Dr Val Hillier in the Computation Department and Baroness McFarlance of Llandaff, Professor of Nursing, both in the Faculty of Medicine at Manchester University, and to Dr P. Hawthorne of Nottingham University.

Finally, my thanks and love must go to my personal support system, especially my husband Eric, whose unfailing support and patience has kept me going, and to my children Tim, Alison and Martin, who have become splendid people in spite of the mistakes their mother made!

1

Birth and change

The birth of a baby is an eagerly awaited event. It is also the beginning of major changes in the life of its parents. Whilst both parents must now undertake new roles and responsibilities, the mother is the one most profoundly affected. Many demands will be made upon her during the period immediately following the birth. During the time of recovery from the physical stress of pregnancy and labour she will experience conflicting emotions of joy and anxiety as she becomes aware of the utter dependence of her infant upon her, and the responsibility which is now hers. She must learn and master new skills in feeding and caring for her baby, and both she and her partner must come to terms with the social restrictions which result from the needs of a new baby. Nor are these transient changes, for this child, and any other children which they may have, will need its parents' care and commitment for many years if his or her full potential as a human being is to be fulfilled.

The birth of a baby is, therefore, not only the beginning of the infant's life; it is also a major life-change bringing about a new pattern of life for the whole family. The pattern which emerges will be influenced by the thoughts, beliefs, personalities and attitude of the people involved, and by the values of the society in which they live.

Any major life-change provokes some degree of stress. Holmes and Rahe (1967) devised a rating scale which lists 43 major life-events in order of the degree of stress with which they are associated. Whilst the death of a spouse is listed as the most stressful life-event, pregnancy and the acquisition of a new family member are both included within the first 20. For some couples a number of other major life-events may be occurring at the same time as pregnancy and the birth of a baby. These may include marriage, changes in financial status, the woman giving up her work, the acquisition of a mortgage, and a change of home. It is small wonder that Brown (1979) described childbirth and the puerperium as uniquely stressful among normal expected life experiences. Becoming a mother makes physical and psychological demands which are complex and severe.

Many women will adapt to motherhood and its demands with a minimum of stress because of their own psychological strengths and the quality of the support they receive from their family and friends. Others will experience severe stress during the transition to motherhood. Some of these will arise from the woman's own psychological needs; others will be caused by external factors such as financial difficulties, a demanding older child, or marital tension. The experience of hospitalisation, too, is stressful to most people, as it causes them to relinquish control over their patterns of daily living. During this time the way in which care is given by professional care-givers should be sensitive and related to individual needs. It should be designed to enhance the mother's particular strengths and confidence, and at the very least should avoid the addition of extra stress by insensitive attitudes or approaches to care. If care-givers are to fulfil this function, they will need to understand something of the psychological processes involved in adjusting to change and coping with stress. The experience of parenting is a mixed blessing and will provoke a number of conflicting reactions and feelings:

> Being a mother is harder work than I had imagined it to be. I now realise that a baby definitely is not a doll to be paraded around in fancy frills!
>
> At times the baby is a real handful and when my husband goes to work after a rough night I feel very depressed and unable to cope. I find that when the baby has been upset all day I am watching the clock and waiting for my husband to come home, and feel relieved when he does.
>
> But when the baby is awake and looking at me and learning to use his arms and legs, or asleep in my arms, I get a feeling of utter peace and contentment and realise he is worth it after all.
>
> Glenis, aged 23, first-time mother

Every individual has a continuing need for physical safety, love and security, esteem and achievement (Maslow 1970). The satisfaction of these needs produces a state of emotional security which can be described as an internal feeling-state of confidence and emotional well-being. The experiences of living involve adapting to numerous changes and many different situations. As a result we develop attitudes and patterns of behaviour which enable us to maintain our state of emotional well-being, and through the development of these patterns we are able to achieve desired objectives, and to develop the maturity to accept disappointment and failure.

When major life-changes occur, or when the normal mechanisms for dealing with change and challenge are not effective, some degree of stress will be experienced until the disturbing situation has been dealt with and overcome. The way in which an individual deals with such a situation has been called the coping process (Lazarus 1969) and is recognised as having a consistent pattern.

Lazarus describes two main forms of demands that are made upon an individual, the interaction of which will form the basis of the way a person reacts to stress. These are the individual's internal needs, which are derived from his or her personality, and learned needs for approval and achievement; and the external demands and expectations of behaviour which are imposed by the values of peers, and the culture to which a person belongs. Lazarus also emphasises that the type of coping behaviour which is adopted by the individual must be understood in terms of a transaction between the individual concerned, the stress being experienced, and the environment in which coping is taking place.

This relationship between the internal and external demands made upon an individual during adjustment to change is taken a stage further by Caplan (1964), who describes three groups of needs which must be met if emotional equilibrium is to be maintained. These are the physical needs of safety, food, shelter etc., the need for personal interaction with others in the family or peer group, and the need to react within the constraints set by the social and cultural mores of the society in which the individual lives.

In all these complex interactions of internal needs and external pressures, strong emotions will be experienced. Emotions are powerful forces which affect perception, understanding, behaviour and attitudes. The effect of emotion will be seen during the period of adjustment to stress and as an end product of the coping process. Nor should it be thought that 'emotions' mean only the weepiness and distress which is often associated with women; emotions also include joy and love, and can be life-enriching and positive. The event of marriage is listed seventh in Holmes and Rahe's list of stressful life-events, and the amount of adjustment required by both partners in a marriage is well recognised. Nevertheless, marriage is usually accompanied by emotions of joy and happiness. Similarly a mother's delight in her child can enable her to overcome considerable physical discomfort and psychological stress.

Women have always sought the help of their female companions during the time of childbirth and mothering, and such records as exist reflect the effect which the culture to which both mother and midwife belonged had upon their relationship with each other. Thus the midwife caring for Rachel during her last and fatal labour, sought to strengthen and encourage her dying patient with the news that she had borne Jacob yet another son, that great status symbol of the Jewish tribe. In more recent years, male-dominated Victorian society, scandalised at the use of chloroform in relieving labour pains because it 'robbed God of the deep and earnest cries of women in the pains of childbirth', had to change its attitudes overnight when Queen Victoria used chloroform for the birth of her eighth child in 1852! Such luxuries were only for the wealthy and influential, however. A remarkable collection of letters from working women which was first published in 1915 gives striking examples of the miseries of childbirth and motherhood endured in poverty and made worse by the 'modesty' which prevented 'respectable' women from seeking help in the prevention of unwanted pregnancies (Llewellyn Davies 1979). These letters were collected as part of a campaign to provide a free midwifery service which would give care to mothers either in their own homes or in local maternity homes.

Midwives and mothers continue to play their complementary roles, even though birth now takes place within the setting of a maternity hospital. Midwives take full responsibility for the labour and delivery of the majority of mothers in the United Kingdom: they run the labour suites, the post-natal wards and the special care baby units; they visit mothers on a daily basis after discharge from hospital for at least ten days after the birth and often for a longer period. It would seem reasonable to suppose, therefore, that the care given to mothers by midwives during this time has an important part to play in enabling women to adjust successfully to the demands which motherhood makes upon them and their families. It is surprising that little attention has been paid to the relationships between mothers and midwives during the crucial first days and weeks following the birth of a baby.

Caplan (1964) considers that people experiencing major upheaval in their lives are more susceptible to the influence of others than they are at times of normal functioning, and that the quality of the support given by others may have the effect of 'loading the dice' in favour of a good or poor outcome. He argues, therefore, that all of the caring professions need to develop their knowledge and technical insight in order to practice more surely the kind of work which will help clients emotionally and mentally, as well as achieving the basic goals of the profession.

If the psychologists are right in their insistence that the outcome of the coping process should be understood in terms of the transaction between the individual, the stress and the environment, then it can be argued that the factor most amenable to change is that of the supportive environment. This approach has been taken by many of the studies of factors affecting the establishment of maternal–child relationships. Klaus and Kennell (1982) suggest that although many of the determinants of parental behaviour are largely permanent, some of them may be changed either favourably or unfavourably during the crisis of birth.

This book is based upon research designed to increase knowledge of the effects which midwives working within the National Health Service may or may not have upon the ability of mothers to adjust to the demands of the post-natal period. The design of the research was based upon the premise that women react to childbirth and motherhood in the same way that people react to any major life-change, and therefore explored the psychological concepts underlying the processes of coping and adjustment in order to identify factors which were likely to affect reactions to motherhood. Previous studies exploring factors related to post-natal depression, and those concerned with factors affecting the development of maternal–child relationships, were also considered, as only when these factors are more fully understood can the role played by the midwife be evaluated.

2

Factors involved in the coping process

Stress and coping

Arnold (1960) defined stress as any condition which disturbs normal functioning. Normal functioning of course varies considerably from person to person according to the factors and events which have contributed to each individual's unique situation. These factors include personality, previous experiences and the particular situation in which stress is being experienced. In addition, normal functioning is often disturbed by an accumulation of small stresses, each of which contributes to the disturbance of normality.

It is vital that care-givers understand that a person's reactions to stress are governed by a multiplicity of internal and external factors, and that although emotions displayed appear to have been provoked by a particular event, they really reflect the results of a complex process many of the features of which are outside the control of either the individual concerned or the care-giver.

Lazarus (1966) describes the way in which people react to and cope with stress in terms of three interacting factors. These are the antecedent factors which predispose the individual's reaction through normal patterns of functioning, the immediate emotional and physical reactions which will initiate the coping response, and the outcome in terms of coping behaviour. Adjustment can be defined as mastery over a situation, and coping as coming to terms with a situation which has not been overcome (Lazarus 1966). The outcome of coping behaviour will be determined by the factors listed above, the degree of stress being experienced, and the quality of the supportive environment surrounding the individual.

Antecedent factors: personality and previous experiences

The main antecedent factors involved in the coping process are personality and previous learning experiences.

Freud (1940) considered that the major facets of personality are fixed before the age of five years and that little change is possible after that age. Other psychologists argue that personality continues to develop from birth onwards, being affected by major changes in the environment and by the learning process. Erikson (1963) describes such changes as developmental crises because of their permanent or semi-permanent effects upon behaviour and thought.

The effect of personality on adjustment to motherhood has been considered by a number of researchers and will be discussed more fully later. Perhaps the most notable study was that by Pitt (1968), on a sample of 305 mothers. He found that 10% of them were depressed six weeks post-partum. Pitt had assessed the personality of the mothers during the last trimester of pregnancy and found that those who had a high anxiety trait formed a significant proportion of those later found to be depressed. Similar effects have been found in the reactions of patients admitted for non-urgent reasons to medical wards. Wilson-Barnett (1979) found that patients with a high anxiety trait took much longer to adjust to the hospital environment than did those with normal or low levels of anxiety.

Previous experiences also influence the coping process. They affect the perception of the situation, the individual's belief in his or her ability to cope, and the motivation needed to adapt to and master the new circumstances.

A very interesting set of studies by Seligman (1975) demonstrated that where subjects were unable to avoid or deal successfully with a stressful situation they tended to slip into apathy and gave up any further attempts to avoid the stress. For them 'taking the punishment' was preferable to further failure at overcoming the painful situation. When the same subjects were later put into a situation in which avoidance and escape were possible, they made no attempt to do either, but accepted the situation and again 'took the punishment'. The prospect of failing yet again was apparently more painful than the stress to which they were subjected, and the key factor appeared to be their belief that they were unable to control the situation in which they were placed. This apathy and lack of motivation to change is described as one form of coping behaviour.

Anxiety

Anxiety may appear at any stage of the coping process, either as an antecedent factor, as a reaction, or as a continuing feature of individual coping behaviour.

There are two main forms of anxiety – trait anxiety and state anxiety – and it is important to realise that both may be operating in a given situation. Trait anxiety is a stable personality trait, whereas state anxiety is a transitory fluctuating response to the perception of danger or threat (Cattell and Scheier 1961). Most people are familiar with some of the physical manifestations of anxiety such as a dry mouth, sweating palms and 'butterflies in the tummy'.

Anxiety affects both perception and understanding. Anxious people are less able to take in information and instruction and tend to blame themselves for their lack of understanding. Midwives may well remember their own reactions of anxiety and distress when becoming a student midwife after working as either a staff nurse or ward sister in general nursing. Many midwives recall the unhappiness and loss of self-esteem which resulted when their previous experience and level of competence were regarded as irrelevant in this new situation. During this period of anxiety they found that the attitude of certain qualified midwives reinforced their feelings of incompetence and further reduced their ability to learn the new skills expected of them. Coping behaviour in this situation usually took the form of avoiding such qualified staff, quickly 'learning the ropes' in order to avoid further stress, and depending very greatly on the support of other students on the same course. The situation which is related by most midwives amply illustrates the primary and secondary reactions to stress described by psychologists and enables us to appreciate both the effects which stress has upon normal functioning, and the way our support systems enable us to overcome stress. Eventually, of course, most student midwives master the new skills expected of them, enabling them in retrospect to laugh at the painful experience. It is notable, however, that very few ever forget it.

Support systems and the supportive environment

'A man does not face crisis alone but is helped or hindered by the people around him, by his family, his friends, neighbourhood, community and nation' (Caplan 1964). Lazarus (1969) also places great emphasis on the need to understand the coping process in the context of the individual's environment. This socio-cultural environment affects the process of coping through its effects upon personality, perception and cognition, and the constraints which its values place upon a person's behaviour. For example, the experience of bereavement is common to all societies, but the expression of grief ranges from the stiff upper lip of the British to the wailing distress of Eastern cultures. It is probable that cultures which allow grief to be expressed and shared help the bereaved person to come to terms with the situation better than those which treat death as an unmentionable subject and thus leave the bereaved person isolated.

Primitive cultures evolved rituals for dealing with the mystery of childbirth which allowed the mother a distinctive role and behaviour model. The support provided for the mother via these rituals is a recognition of her needs and her society's understanding that the joys and fears of childbirth should not be faced alone but shared by a supportive group. Kitzinger (1978) explored present-day birth rituals in both developed and less developed countries and concluded that all maternal behaviour is a direct response to the attitudes of the society in which she lives.

The supportive environment, therefore, can be seen to have some role to play in influencing a person's adjustment to change and stress. In fact if the antecedent factors which will predispose the coping reaction are permanent or semi-permanent features of an individual's make-up, then the only variable factor in the coping process is that of the environment in which change is being faced. This has been highlighted in various studies into the factors affecting maternal–child relationships in the early post-natal period. Klaus and Kennell (1970, 1976, 1982) demonstrated that the attitudes and practices of hospital staff could be changed in order to provide an environment which enhanced rather than hindered the attachment process between mother and baby.

The term 'support' is freely used in nursing and medical reports, but its meaning in relation to the individual patient is often not defined. Caplan (Caplan and Killilea 1976) defines support as 'an enduring pattern of continuous or intermittent ties that play a significant part in maintaining the psychological and physical integrity of the individual over time'. Whilst the support provided for an individual by his or her family is of paramount importance, that offered by peer, friend, professional helpers and social institutions may also make a considerable difference to emotional well-being and coping ability. Weiss (1976) defines effective support as that given by a person, either professional or lay, who is accepted as an ally by the distressed person. The helper's acceptance will depend upon the ability to convince the distressed person that his or her training and experience, understanding and commitment are available for as long as they are needed. This in turn will depend upon a two-way exchange of information and mutual trust, and the development of a relationship between the helper and the person needing help. The role of the helper is to listen as well as to instruct, and to give help which is relevant to the needs of the individual rather than in compliance with a preconceived model of how that person should react.

When considering the role of support systems in the adjustment of women to childbirth and motherhood, it is interesting to note that many studies in this area have either concentrated upon factors in the mother which are related to post-natal depression without considering her environment, or have criticised the hospital environment without considering the factors in the mother which are related to post-natal depression or would have affected her reaction to hospitalisation. Oakley (1980) believes that many studies on transition to motherhood have suffered from their disregard of the socio-cultural context surrounding childbirth.

The growth among mothers of self-help groups such as the National Childbirth Trust and the La Leche League may be indications of the failure of family or professional helpers to provide

appropriate support. They illustrate that relationship between
the helper and the individual being helped that is described by
Weiss. They also exert an influence upon the mother's behaviour
by their values and the emphasis placed upon certain aspects
of motherhood such as breast feeding. This may lead to their
membership mainly consisting of women with similar attitudes
and values, but their success nevertheless amply illustrates the
value of an acceptable and appropriate support system.

An understanding of the role which a support system may
have in influencing the outcome of the coping process leads to
a realisation that no set pattern or routine provision can meet
the needs of all individuals. Whilst the initial reaction to stress
will be profoundly affected by the fixed antecedent factors of
personality, previous experiences and expectations, the professional helper can influence the situation by the appropriateness
of the help provided. Such help should therefore be flexible in
its approach and degree.

The support system surrounding women during pregnancy,
labour and childbirth consists of family and peers, and the maternity services provided by the society in which the woman lives.
In the United Kingdom this service is given via the National
Health Service and spans care given by general practitioners,
midwives and health visitors in the primary care team, and
obstetricians, paediatricians, midwives, anaesthetists and
physiotherapists in the hospital services.

The developments in medicine and technology designed to
reduce perinatal and maternal mortality have mainly taken place
during the last thirty years, and have thereby changed social
and family patterns of support for childbirth which had been
in existence for many centuries. In the United Kingdom 99%
of all births now take place in hospitals or GP maternity units.
Among other things this means that for many women their first
experience of hospitalisation coincides with the experience of
childbirth and motherhood. There is a danger that those of us
who spend our working lives in the hospital environment may
not appreciate the stress which admission to hospital and the
loss of control over patterns of daily living can cause to patients.

The manner in which maternity care is provided has been
the focus of discussion in recent years, and the report of the
Social Services Committee on Perinatal and Maternal Mortality

(Great Britain 1980) pointed out that the emotional support given to mothers was of major importance. It went on to say that any mother who produced a healthy baby but looked back on the experience as one she would not want to repeat should be regarded as evidence of failure of the service!

Understanding the outcome of coping behaviour

The type of coping behaviour which results from any stressful change or situation will be relevant to the individual's internal needs and provide the most appropriate way of dealing with the situation. Lazarus (1966) describes four main forms of coping behaviour, all of which are designed to enable the person concerned to cope with a stressful situation which is not yet overcome. These are:

Anticipatory action
Attack
Avoidance
Apathy and inaction

Anticipatory action

Anticipatory action can be seen in the fevered study undertaken by some students as the day of an examination draws near. Such students have been found to be extremely sensitive to any clue which might assist their preparations and indicate the likely question they will be expected to answer (Mechanic 1962). A similar form of anticipatory action underlies the belief held by professionals and mothers that ante-natal classes in preparation for childbirth and mothering enable the mother to cope – but such classes need to be related to the mother's real needs. Perkins (1979) found that attendance at such classes was related to the mother's social class and the degree to which she considered the teaching relevant to her situation. Mothers who had been dissatisfied with the classes later dismissed them as being of no use in coping with labour and delivery. Mothers of lower social class did not attend and the reasons given were that they did not know what to expect.

Another example of anticipatory action is the wide range of books on pregnancy and baby care, and the amount of literature produced by the Health Education Council. This brings into question the validity of much that is produced and the expectations thus aroused. Recent publications which are honest in their descriptions of some of the frustrations and stresses which may be experienced alongside the joys and delights are to be welcomed. By exploring and giving credence to the wide variety of reactions of mothers and babies they can reduce the feelings of failure and guilt which unreal presentations of 'ideal mothers' and 'model' babies may produce.

Anticipatory action also occurs in the body's psychological response to danger or the threat of danger, and in behavioural reactions. Shannon and Isbell (1963) found that military personnel who were anticipating painful dentistry produced the same psychological reaction of adrenaline release at the expectation of an injection as did those who actually received the injection. A person's understanding of a situation has also been shown to affect physiological and behavioural reactions. Janis (1958) found that the intensity of fear and anxiety in patients awaiting surgery was not related to the seriousness of the surgery, but to their understanding of the processes involved. Hayward (1975) found that stress could be reduced by giving appropriate information to patients before surgery, and that the amount of post-operative pain reported by patients who had received such information was considerably reduced. This was confirmed by the fact of a reduction in the amount of post-operative pain relief required.

Whilst the results of such studies may justify the use of ante-natal classes in preparing women for the stresses of labour and delivery, they also highlight the need for information to be relevant and appropriate to the woman concerned. They underline too the need to understand the fear which may be aroused when women are admitted in labour into stark clinical surroundings in a labour ward. If the atmosphere of a delivery suite is reminiscent of an operating theatre, a visit paid to it during ante-natal classes may arouse more fear than it seeks to allay. The recent development of delivery rooms which look like ordinary bedrooms, the use of reduced lighting and the presence of the woman's husband or other companion during labour are to be welcomed in reducing the fear which strange and threatening situations may arouse.

Attack

The purpose of attack as a means of coping with stress is to demolish or destroy the agent or situation which is provoking (or is perceived as provoking) the stress. Attack may be verbal or physical, and the means of expressing it will be constrained by social and cultural values. It is regarded by many as an instinctive action, and Freud (1957) considered that war could be seen as an inevitable expression of such an instinct. As a way of coping with unacceptable stress it usually has to be succeeded by other ways of dealing with the situation.

The mother who insists upon a rigid routine of baby care and household chores to which she, her husband and children must conform, may also be using attack as a means of coping with a situation which she fears may overwhelm her if allowed to slip out of her control. Likewise the existence and activities of certain pressure groups that want to change the present patterns of maternity care may arise from the stresses produced in their members during pregnancy and childbirth. While most such groups make informed and constructive criticisms of the professionals concerned, attack as a form of coping may be seen in the consistently destructive criticism expressed by certain individuals.

Avoidance

Another form of coping behaviour is avoidance of any situation which invokes painful memories of previous stress. Students may find plausible excuses for dropping a difficult course of study; children may run away from an unhappy home. The large number of people who 'disappear' every year, leaving behind their homes, families and livelihood also illustrates avoidance behaviour. Suicide can be seen as avoidance behaviour in its most extreme form, and agoraphobia as avoidance of the fear-provoking world outside the safe home environment.

The 'learned helplessness' found by Seligman (1975) showed that vulnerable animals and human beings preferred to accept a painful situation rather than experience the pain of failure once again. They avoided making the effort to get out of the painful situation because the recurrence of failure would form a greater threat to their self-esteem. The reluctance of some women to attend ante-natal clinics in hospital may not be a rejection of the expertise offered at such clinics, but avoidance of the stress incurred by the difficulties of making a long journey to the hospital, coping with older children during the visit, or the experience of being deprived of personal clothing and identity as they pass along the ante-natal clinic conveyor belt. All of these factors may combine to make non-attendance an appropriate form of coping.

Avoidance behaviour may have physiological as well as psychological effects, and stress has been recognised as a significant contributory factor in heart disease.

Apathy and inaction

Continuing patterns of being unable to overcome a stressful situation can lead to persistent apathy and inaction. Coping with stress may have physiological as well as psychological effects. Stress has been recognised as a contributory factor in the formation of stomach ulcers and in heart disease.

This was uniquely demonstrated by the 'executive monkey' experiment (Brady *et al.* 1958). This experiment was set up to examine the reaction to physiological stress in two monkeys which were restrained in chairs through which they received a brief electric shock at twenty-second intervals. One monkey (the executive monkey) was able to prevent the shock to both himself and his partner by learning to press a lever just before the shock was due. He therefore had to cope with learning to use the lever and with learning to press it at the right time. Failure resulted in a shock being received by both. The second monkey had no means itself of preventing the shock but was totally dependent on its partner's ability.

The executive monkey developed stomach ulcers as a response to stress, whilst the non-executive did not, but became apathetic and depressed in the face of his inability to exert any control over his situation. It was initially considered that the effort required of the executive monkey in taking repeated appropriate action in order to avoid the painful electric shock was more stressful than the shock itself. However, this conclusion was changed when the non-executive monkey died unexpectedly of a heart attack. Whilst both the ulcers and the heart attack developed as a result of the stresses incurred, it could be argued that the heart attack removed the non-executive monkey from his intolerable situation, thus taking avoidance behaviour to its ultimate degree.

The behaviour of the non-executive monkey demonstrates the fourth form of coping cited by Lazarus, that of apathy and inaction. It is seen when a person believes there is no hope of either avoidance or attack. Lazarus defines inaction as 'the complete absence of any impulse to deal with a situation' and cites Mintz's (1951) description of the lack of panic seen when people are trapped with no means of escape, such as in a submarine or mining disaster. Hilgard, Atkinson and Atkinson (1979) give the example of concentration camp victims for whom apathy and inaction had become such a persistent behavioural pattern that they were totally unable to respond to their liberation by allied troops at the end of the war. Increased understanding of the causes of apathy and inaction may help midwives understand and respond to mothers with multiple social problems who do not seek help until pregnancy is well advanced or until labour itself begins.

Apathy and inaction can be seen as symptoms of depression (Lazarus 1966). Dalton (1980) describes depression as a disease of loss, characterised by gloom, despondency and despair. Victims of depression experience the loss of happiness, pleasure, interest and enthusiasm, as well as the ability to think clearly, to concentrate or to remember. Other losses may include appetite, sleep, weight control and bowel movement.

Post-natal depression is one end of a whole spectrum of emotional reactions to motherhood. At the other end is the happy, fulfilled and well-adjusted mother who delights in her new status and role. In between are the majority of women who calmly adjust to motherhood without experiencing the euphoria of one extreme or the depression of the other.

Summary

This brief exploration of some of the concepts of the coping process and support system indicate that:
1. Personality and previous experience are powerful antecedent factors which predispose a person's reaction to change.
2. The coping behaviour shown by an individual is relevant to the needs of that individual and is not a matter for judgement or approval.

3. The person experiencing stress can be helped by someone whose unconditional support is available to them, and who understands something of the situation and the factors involved in the coping process.

3

Emotional reactions to motherhood, maternal–child relationships and post-natal care

Studies of the way women react and adjust to motherhood fall into two main categories: those concerned with factors relating to post-natal depression, and those concerned with the establishment of maternal–child relationships.

Emotional reactions to motherhood

Emotional reactions to the experience of childbirth and mothering range from those mothers (and fathers) who are very happy and well adjusted, to those for whom the experience produces depression and despondency. Post-natal depression is unique in that it can only start after a pregnancy, and has other features which distinguish it from 'typical' depression in adults. Irritability is a common feature of post-natal depression and disturbances of sleep patterns varies from that in other forms of depression. Most patients with depression may get off to sleep successfully but then find that they wake early and cannot get back to sleep. Women with post-natal depression, however, have a great need of sleep and seem unable to get enough. They sleep heavily, waking only to attend to the baby, and can then sleep through the day if they have the opportunity. Most depressed patients dread the mornings, but post-natally depressed mothers are at their best in the morning and feel progressively worse as the day goes on (Dalton 1980).

Pitt (1968) described the symptoms of the 'atypical' depression of the post-natal period as tearfulness, despondency, feelings of inadequacy and an inability to cope, together with guilt linked to self-reproach about not loving or caring properly for the baby. These feelings were almost always accompanied by anxiety about the baby, even though all the babies in the study were thriving.

Certain studies have sought to explain women's adaptation to motherhood in terms of their 'femininity'. In a descriptive study of maternal emotions, Newton (1955) explored the feelings of mothers towards menstruation, pregnancy and childbirth, breast feeding, care of the infant and 'other aspects of their femininity'. Chertok (1969) and Nilsson (1972) both produced scales of 'femininity' from which they attempted to show that post-natal depression was related to a woman's rejection of her feminine role in childbirth. One wonders what the reaction might be if it were suggested that depression occurring in men following trauma was due to some default in their 'masculinity'.

The majority of studies of post-natal depression, however, can be related to the concepts of the coping process, with depression being considered as the result of the interaction of various factors.

In a study of 700 pregnancies Tod (1964) found that 3% of the mothers suffered from post-natal depression of sufficient severity to require psychiatric help. All the depressed mothers had shown marked anxiety during the pregnancy, while abnormal obstetric history, poor family and social background, and what Tod described as 'inadequate' personality, all contributed to the incidence of depression. He concluded that post-natal depression was the end result of long-established maladjustment and should not be regarded as a specific disorder of the puerperium.

A comprehensive study by Pitt (1968) found that 10% of a random sample of 305 women were depressed post-partum. The study was based on an interview and questionnaire which explored depressive symptoms in the women. The questionnaire was completed during the last trimester of pregnancy and again six to eight weeks after the birth of the baby. Pitt also used the Maudsley Medical Inventory (Eysenck 1959) to assess personality during the last trimester. He found that depression in the puerperium was not related to parity nor to the events of labour and delivery. The most marked finding was the relationship of a high anxiety trait score on the Maudsley Medical Inventory to the incidence of depression in the puerperium. The depressed mothers expressed feelings of despondency, inadequacy and an inability to cope, especially with the baby. The depression was most marked on their return home from the hospital. Mothers complained of undue fatigue and sleep disturbance over and above that to be expected from the demands of a small infant. One of the more disturbing features of this study was that 43% of the depressed mothers had not improved when followed up a year later! Pitt concluded that there was a large pool of generally unrecognised emotional distress in women during the puerperium.

Dewi-Rees and Lutkin (1971) also found 10% of 91 mothers and 77 fathers were depressed both before and after childbirth, which adds weight to Pitt's contention that there is a large pool of emotional distress in mothers during the puerperium. The evidence that fathers also suffer stress due to life-crisis change further discredits the theory of 'maladjusted femininity' as a cause of post-natal depression. Unfortunately, as this study was undertaken mainly to assess the usefulness of the Beck Depression Inventory in identifying depression among patients in general practice, very little detail is given about other factors which were related to the depression identified.

Dalton (1971) found that 7% of a sample of 189 mothers were depressed following childbirth. The depressed women were predominantly those who had expressed a high degree of welcome for the pregnancy and an eagerness to breast feed. Tod and Dewi-Rees and Dalton all found evidence of labile emotions during pregnancy in women who were subsequently depressed. Dalton argues from earlier work (Dalton 1964) that maladjustment to the hormonal changes in the puerperium is a major precipitating factor in women who are vulnerable to post-natal depression. Hormonal changes are frequently presented as the cause of 'third day blues' and Dalton places strong emphasis on their effect. Studies of continuing depression, however, suggest that third day blues are a transitory feature, and that continuing depressed mood is related to other, more long-standing factors.

A study by Frommer and O'Shea (1973) considered the effect of maternal deprivation upon mothering outcome. By use of a simple questioning schedule in the ante-natal clinic they were able to identify women who had been separated from one or both of their parents before the age of 11 years. They found 58 women who reported separation, and matched them with 58 others who had not been thus separated. It was found that women in the separated group had a higher incidence of depression and were much more anxious about their babies than those in the non-separated group. In addition, they found that when difficulties arose with the care or well-being of their infants, mothers in the separated group were much more distressed and anxious than the other women. Frommer and O'Shea concluded that evidence of separation from parents during childhood could be used by midwives and health visitors to identify vulnerable women.

Brown and Harris (1978) found that separation from both parents before the age of 11 years was also a feature of the history of depressed women as a whole, and not just of post-natally depressed women. Vulnerability to depression was related to low social class, the lack of a confiding and warm relationship with the husband or male partner, separation from parents before the age of 11, and having three or more children under the age of 5 years. In other words, an interaction of antecedent factors and life-crisis stress resulted in apathy and depression.

A study by Kumar and Robson (1978) used the Eysenck Personality Inventory (EPI) to assess the relationship of maternal personality and emotional status during pregnancy and again three months after delivery. The Social Readjustment Rating Scale (Holmes and Rahe 1967) was used to identify concurrent life-crises and the emotional well-being of the mothers was assessed by the Standardised Psychiatric Interview (Goldberg *et al.* 1974) Kumar and Robson found that 19 of their sample of 119 primiparae were depressed three months after delivery (16%) and that the depression was related to marital tension, difficult relationships within the family situation, original doubts about the pregnancy and a history of infertility. They did not find that depression three months after delivery was related to anxiety trait measured on the EPI. But in a prospective study throughout the pregnancy of the mothers in the sample Kumar and Robson found that high anxiety trait measured on the EPI was related to depression during the first trimester of pregnancy, to marital tension and to a history of previous termination of pregnancy. In six mothers depression during the second and third trimesters was related to life-crisis events of bereavements and illness of a close family member.

Cox (1978) studied a group of 186 Ugandan women during

pregnancy and until the puerperium, and found that 9.7% of them suffered post-natal depression. The symptoms described by the women were very similar to those in Pitt's study and Cox concludes that psychiatric morbidity in any group of women must be understood in relation to socio-cultural factors.

These studies illustrate the complexity of factors which affect the emotional well-being of women during pregnancy and childbirth, and it is notable that only one of them found that obstetric history was a factor in subsequent depression. Personality, marital stress and other life-crises had a strong relationship with emotional outcome.

A sociologically based study of 55 women by Oakley (1980) explored a number of influences on transition to motherhood. The women were studied from the twenty-eighth week of pregnancy until five months after the birth. Four measures of mental health and two measures of satisfaction with motherhood were used. The four measures of mental health were post-natal blues during hospitalisation, anxiety about the baby, depressed moods occurring after the first three weeks of the puerperium, and depression. Depression was defined as a depressed state occurring at any time between discharge from hospital and five months post-partum. The mother's satisfaction with motherhood was assessed in terms of self-reports of her feelings about the role of mothering and its skills, and her strength of positive and negative feelings about the baby.

Oakley found that early post-natal blues were associated with dissatisfaction about the conduct of the second stage of labour and with epidural analgesia. Mothers in social classes 4 and 5 were more likely to suffer depressed moods and depression was linked to marital tension and poor housing. Low satisfaction with motherhood was linked to poor support and low self-image. The study thus revealed a number of factors likely to produce anxiety and depression in any group of people, underlining once again that depression following the birth of a baby is associated with normal patterns of stress and coping.

In an earlier study of the emotional needs of mothers (Ball 1981), 178 women completed a questionnaire about their satisfaction with the care they had received, and about their own feelings six weeks after the birth. Differences were found between those women who were classed as having high emotional well-being and those classed as being emotionally distressed. These differences were social class, the degree of satisfaction with post-natal care, and the mother's report of her feelings immediately after the birth of her baby. Mothers in social class 4 scored lower levels of satisfaction with all aspects of their maternity care and formed the largest proportion of the emotionally distressed group. Dissatisfaction with post-natal care was associated with marked anxiety about the baby and the incidence of conflicting advice from midwives. There was also some evidence of a relationship between the mother's emotional state six weeks post-partum and her reported feelings immediately after the birth. However, as this report was obtained six weeks after the birth it is likely that the mother's emotional state at that time would have affected her perception of the birth.

These studies of factors related to differences in post-natal emotional well-being in women confirm that personality and previous experiences affect adjustment to motherhood, and that additional stresses arising from marital tension and other life-crises have a detrimental effect upon the adjustment process.

Maternal–child relationships

The post-natal period does not only mark the end of a pregnancy, but more importantly the beginning (or continuation in a more substantial form) of the relationship between the mother and her infant. In recent years a growing volume of research has focused upon these relationships and the effect which the supportive environment may have upon their establishment and continuing development.

Bowlby's (1951, 1961) work on the effects of contemporary methods of child care on the psychological well-being of the child led him to the conclusion that a warm, continuing relationship between the child and its mother, or a permanent mother substitute, was essential. The results of Bowlby's work were to revolutionise attitudes to and organisation of the care of children in institutions and to affect profoundly the work of the child-caring professions.

More recently the work of Klaus and Kennell (1970, 1976, 1982) and their associates has been of major influence (Klaus *et al.* 1972; Kennell *et al.* 1974; Hales *et al.* 1977). They present evidence that the first hour following birth is a particularly sensitive period in the establishment of close ties between parents and their infant. They found that when a mother is left alone with her baby she will follow a particular pattern of exploration of her baby's body, and that this exploration can be interrupted by the presence of a third person other than the father. Eye contact between the parents and child has been shown to be of particular significance, and when an infant is held at the breast to suckle, this provides the ideal *en face* position for eye contact to take place. Whilst the sensitive period is believed to be particularly important, Klaus and Kennell and their colleagues (Klaus and Kennell 1982) also point out that the relationship between mother and infant is one which grows and develops over the days and weeks, and can be fostered by easy and regular contact between mother (and father) and infant. They also emphasise that the amount of time that mothers and babies spend together in the early days after birth should be controlled by the mother, and that the constant presence of a demanding baby may be detrimental in the short term to the relationship with the mother.

The claims made for a sensitive period in human mothers (Kennell, Trause and Klaus 1975) have been criticised, and a later publication by Klaus and Kennell (1982) takes note of these criticisms. Dunn and Richard (1977) found that the choice of method of feeding and the birth order of the infant have an effect upon the type of mother–infant interaction which takes place immediately after delivery and during the first ten days of the infant's life.

Klaus and Kennell (1976, 1982) define two main groups of factors which impinge upon the establishment of maternal–child relationships. One group relates to factors in the mother, such as her personality, culture and family relationships; the other relates to factors in the caring environment, such as the attitudes and practices of doctors and midwives, and the policies of the hospital in such matters as the avoidance of separation during the post-natal period.

Factors in the mother's personality and previous experience have already been discussed in connection with post-natal depression. In Frommer and O'Shea's study (1973) it was found that where a mother had been separated from her parents before the age of 11, and was also experiencing difficulties in her relationship with the baby's father, her difficulties in mothering were considerably increased. Stott (1962, 1973) considered that child morbidity and behavioural problems were much more common in the offspring of women who had difficulties in their relationships with other people, both inside and outside the family. Broussard and Hartner (1971) found that the mothers whose self-concept was poor and whose degree of self-esteem was low were more likely to see their babies as difficult, and they were observed to have continuing difficulties with their babies.

Lynch, Roberts and Gordon (1976) found that mothers whose infant had been placed on the 'at risk' non-accidental injury register suffered from diffuse problems in personal relationships. They also found that such mothers had been noted by the midwives caring for them in the immediate post-natal period in hospital, and that midwives had observed at that time that the mothers were having some difficulty in mothering their infants. Another study of women who abused their babies (Rosen and Stein 1980) found that the women concerned had low self-esteem and had previously experienced difficulty with close relationships.

The events of pregnancy are also said to have an effect upon the maternal–child relationship. Ferreira (1960), in a longitudinal study of women during pregnancy and after delivery, found that the babies of mothers who had been classed as highly anxious during pregnancy cried more frequently and for longer periods than the babies of less anxious mothers. He concluded that this was due to pre-natal influences rather than post-natal mismanagement. Another study (Wolkind 1981) indicated that there was a relationship between psychiatric disturbance in the mother during pregnancy and subsequent low birth weight of the infant.

Provision for the care of mothers during childbirth and the puerperium

The evidence from studies of post-natal depression and the development of maternal–child relationships confirms that reactions to the experience of motherhood vary considerably, and that a number of factors in the mother can be identified as affecting adjustment to motherhood. The supportive environment within which change is taking place also has an effect upon the coping mechanism. The most influential source of support is the family and friends of the individual concerned, but professional care-givers have a role to play as well, and the attitudes and values of society also affect support systems (Caplan 1964, 1969; Caplan and Killilea 1976). Caplan maintains that the actions and attitudes of professional care-givers can be used to 'load the dice' in favour of a good or bad outcome.

Until the latter half of the twentieth century women gave birth at home, receiving what help was available. For many women this care was inadequate and unskilled (Llewellyn Davies 1979); for others, medical staff provided a modicum of expertise. The provision of skilled care for women in childbirth has developed rapidly in this century and one of the major changes has been the replacement of home by the hospital as the usual place for birth to take place. This has the effect of changing long-standing social and family patterns of support, and the discontent expressed by a number of pressure groups indicates that the emotional needs of mothers and babies have been overlooked in the process. More recent years have seen a marked swing towards 'humanising' the system, especially in labour wards.

Pitt (1968) considered that because his study showed that post-natal depression was not related to either parity or obstetric history, the effect of hospital delivery upon emotional outcome was probably irrelevant. Other studies, however, indicate that admission to hospital provokes its own particular stress, and as the majority of women are now delivered in hospital the impact of hospital admission cannot be ignored.

One of the difficulties appears to be the tendency to regard everyone admitted to hospital as a patient, thereby adopting a sickness concept which is inappropriate to the normal physiological process of childbirth. It also overlooks the fact that the birth of a new human being is an intensely personal, emotional and family-centred event.

Studies of reactions to hospital admission indicate that patients do not undervalue the treatment and care that they receive, but are made anxious by, and dislike, the strangeness of the hospital environment. Topliss (1970) found that one of the major reasons why women preferred to give birth at home was their dislike of the hospital atmosphere and its rules. Totman (1979) described the orderly hospital environment as one which requires the subordination of the patient's real world persona and the learning of a highly specialised structure of relationships in which the role of the patient is firmly defined and controlled by the professional staff. Studies by Hayward (1975) and Wilson-Barnett (1979) both illustrate the effects of hospital admission on the patient's understanding and anxiety levels.

Hayward found that the giving of specific information about what to expect after surgery reduced post-operative pain and that patients who received this information required less pain relief than others who had been 'chatted' to for the same amount of time but had not been given specific information or an opportunity to discuss their fears and ask questions. Wilson-Barnett used the Eysenck Personality Inventory to assess trait anxiety in patients admitted for non-urgent medical conditions on the day of their admission to hospital. She then used Lishman's Mood Adjective list to assess state anxiety levels on each day the patient spent in hospital after admission. This revealed a high level of anxiety in all patients on the day of admission, and in patients with high anxiety trait she found that this anxiety did not subside until five days after admission. During this time the degree of anxiety being experienced would reduce the patient's ability to take in any information which was given.

It is unlikely that any great trend away from hospital delivery will develop in the United Kingdom and the Short Report (Great Britain 1980) emphasised that 'humanising' the system would go a long way towards making hospital care more acceptable to the majority of women.

The trend towards hospital delivery for all infants began in the 1960s and was accelerated by the Peel Report (Great Britain 1970). In 1983 99% of all births took place in a hospital or general practitioner maternity unit (Great Britain 1982).

One of the early effects of increasing the number of hospital deliveries was the need either to provide more post-natal beds or to send mothers and babies home to the community midwife's care before the tenth day of the puerperium. (Before 1960 it was usual for women delivered in hospital to remain there for at least 10 days.) Community midwives at this time were a completely separate service caring for the women they had delivered at home. In Bradford (Theobald 1959) an experiment began which rapidly became the norm throughout the country, in which women who were delivered in hospital were transferred home at around 48 hours after delivery. This had a number of organisational results. Mothers are usually asked during the ante-natal period about the length of time they would prefer to stay in hospital after the birth, and these arrangements are then confirmed by the community midwife who will undertake the mother's care. This has the effect of reinforcing in the mother's mind that she has booked for 48 hours irrespective of any change which might be required due to the events of labour or delivery, and any change which does occur in the arrangements causes considerable distress.

These arrangements for discharge early in the puerperium led to a number of agreements being drawn up between hospital and community midwives about the various tasks each would perform on behalf of the mother. Generally, if a mother was booked for a 48-hour stay the hospital staff would initiate feeding and show her how to provide some daily care for her infant, while the major part of educating and supporting the mother in her care of her baby would be undertaken by the community midwife. This tended to develop a chronological approach to the amount of care the mother received and the amount of care she was expected to give to her baby, irrespective of other needs she might have or her degree of experience in infant care. Another effect was the routine physical examination of the mother by a junior houseman on the day after delivery. At this examination the mother would be pronounced 'fit' to go home, ignoring the fact that physical and emotional recovery is a gradual process which takes place throughout the six weeks of the puerperium and beyond it, and is related to each woman's physical and psychological status.

The period of 48 hours after delivery as the optimum time for discharge home was chosen as an administratively convenient time period in which to make suitable arrangements and to allow the mother some rest after the birth. Its effect has been to fragment post-natal care at around the 'third day' crisis, when the euphoria of the birth has passed and the greatness of the responsibility for caring for this new human being has become clear to its parents. It has also tended to reinforce the concept or myth of the 'normal' mother. Thus it is expected that 'most' mothers can undertake full responsibility for the care of their babies on the day after delivery, and 'should' be able to cope fully with infant feeding in the first few days after the birth. Our concepts of 'normal' or 'average' are determined to a large degree by our own culture and class consciousness, and may be inappropriate to the real needs of a widely differing population of mothers. Bronfenbrenner (1958) found that attitudes to childbearing and parenting are constantly changing and that such changes are led by middle class attitudes. Working class parents may, therefore, be 'out of fashion' or may reject middle class concepts entirely.

The value judgements of doctors and midwives also affect the way in which care is given. Routine-centred patterns of care in which the midwife who 'gets the work done' is valued can lead to intensive procedures and insufficient time being spent with an inexperienced or anxious mother (Ball and Stanley 1984; Laryea (1984). McKeith (1966) maintained that the overriding principle in helping a mother adapt to her new infant was that of encouragement and praise and that any suggestion of failure (i.e. not conforming to expectations of the 'normal' mother) was threatening to the mother's self-image and to her relationship with her baby. Curry (1982) declares that helping a mother proceed at her own pace would take more time not less, but should be the aim of all who care for mothers and their newborn infants.

If midwives and other members of the obstetric team are to fulfil the role of helper described by Caplan and Weiss, they will need to recognise factors which affect the emotional needs of women and their babies, and plan the kind of post-natal care which will best meet those needs and result in a strengthening of the woman's emotional well-being. At best, midwives are in a position to enhance and enrich the experience of motherhood; at worst they should not cause any extra stress to a mother because of their lack of understanding of the psychological processes involved.

There is ample evidence that certain factors which affect

adjustment can be identified, and it should be possible to use this information in the planning of appropriate models of care. There is little evidence available concerning the effect which current patterns of post-natal care has upon the maternal adjustment process (Pitt 1978). The research described in this book investigated a number of factors in the mother which would be likely to affect her reactions, and considered their effect alongside those which the nature of the post-natal care given by midwives had upon maternal emotional well-being and satisfaction with motherhood six weeks after the birth of the infant.

4

Undertaking the research

In view of the issues which arise from a review of the many and varied factors involved in adjusting to motherhood, the question to which the research addressed itself was:

> Given the many internal and external factors which affect the way women respond to the psychological, physical and family changes which follow the birth of a child, what effect, if any, do the current patterns of care provided by the midwifery services of the National Health Service have upon this process of adaptation?

The research was designed as a descriptive study of the experiences and reactions of women during childbirth and the first six weeks of their infant's life, as they coped with and adapted to the demands which the birth of their infant made upon them and upon their families. It was a mainly prospective study in terms of the events of labour and post-natal care and the assessment of emotional well-being in the mother six weeks after delivery, but also contained retrospective elements in the mother's assessment of labour and the post-natal care she had received.

The research method was based upon a descriptive survey methodology described by Oppenheim (1966) as an analytic and relational survey. It was designed to allow statistical analysis by computer.

Descriptive surveys are usually based upon a representative sample of the target population in order that the findings may be generalised to the population as a whole. It was not possible, within the constraints of time and finance, to base this survey upon such a representative sample. Instead, a cohort group of women in late pregnancy were studied who were booked for delivery in one of three maternity hospitals. They were included in the research from approximately the thirty-sixth week of pregnancy until six weeks after the birth of the baby.

The target population was defined as pregnant women booked for delivery in Consultant Maternity Hospitals in England during 1981 and 1982. The three hospitals selected were each in a different part of the country. Hospital 1 was a large hospital sited in a cathedral city and serving a wide urban and rural population. Hospital 2 was a smaller hospital in an industrial town in the Midlands, serving mainly a mining and industrial community. Hospital 3 was a professorial unit which had a number of regional sub-specialities and served women from a wide range of other health authorities as well as its own inner city population.

In order to achieve a sample sufficiently large to allow the effects of post-natal care to be differentiated from other factors involved in emotional well-being it was decided to aim for a sample of 100 women in each hospital. The target recruitment number in each hospital was then set at 120 to allow for wastage due to non-response.

Selection of women for the study
Participants were selected from the ante-natal records of women who were due to give birth during the three months of the study. In order to avoid a number of extraneous variables which might affect maternal perceptions of pregnancy, birth and puerperium, the following categories of women were excluded from the selection process:
1. Women with a history of infertility leading up to the current pregnancy.
2. Women who had suffered stillbirth or neonatal death in a previous pregnancy; those who had required admission to an ante-natal word before the thirty-sixth week of their current pregnancy; women with diabetes or other known medical complications; women with known multiple pregnancy.
3. Women from Asian communities were excluded because of language difficulties and different cultural attitudes. West Indian women who had been born in the United Kingdom were included; those born in the West Indies were excluded.

4. Mothers aged under 16 years of age or over 40 years.
5. Mothers whose babies were to be adopted.

Recruitment

The total number of women recruited and for whom full data were obtained is shown in Table 4.1. It can be seen that a smaller number of women were recruited in hospital 3. This was due to severe weather in the winter of 1981, during which many mothers did not attend the ante-natal clinic.

Age groups of the participants

The age groups of the women in the final sample were as follows:

Under 20 years	31 (11.1%)
21–29 years	164 (58.8%)
30–39 years	84 (30.1%)

There was no statistically significant difference in the distribution of age groups across the three hospitals (chi-square = 1.33593 with 4 d.f. P = 0.9553).

Parity of the participants

Ninety-eight of the women (35.4%) were primagravidae, 118 (42.3%) were having their second baby, 38 (13.6%) were having their third baby, and the remaining 25 (9%) were having a fourth child. One set of twins is included in the final sample; these were born to a primigravid woman of 19 years of age.

Social class and marital status of the participants

There was a wide spread of social class in the sample, as can be seen from Table 4.2. There was a significant difference in the

Table 4.1 *Numbers of mothers recruited and interviewed, final sample and response rate*

	Hospital 1	Hospital 2	Hospital 3	Total sample
Mothers recruited	122	127	98	347
Interviewed after delivery	117	119	84	320
Returned post-natal questionnaire	112	104	63	279
Response rate of mothers interviewed after delivery	95.7%	87.3%	75.0%	87.0%

distribution of social class of the sample between the three hospitals (chi-square = 31.08387 with 12 d.f.; P = 0.0019). Hospital 1 had the highest proportion of mothers from social classes 1 and 2, and hospital 3 had the highest proportion of mothers from social class 5.

Twenty-nine of the mothers were single (10.4%), 5 were separated or divorced (1.8%) and the majority (245; 87.8%) were married and living with their spouse.

Choice of hospitals
The three hospitals were selected because each was operating a slightly different method of organising post-natal care. In all three the majority of mothers and babies went home around 48 hours after delivery, and all the hospitals were midwifery training schools.

Hospital 1 had 101 beds, and 4040 births during 1981. In this district all mothers booked for hospital delivery were visited by their community midwife at least three times during pregnancy, and for at least 28 days after the birth.

Hospital 2 had 52 beds, and 2600 births during 1981. There was no regular pattern of visiting the mother at home during pregnancy, and mothers were visited daily for at least 10 days after delivery. When the midwife considered it necessary the visits were extended beyond 10 days and up to 28 days.

Hospital 3 had 149 beds, and 4500 births during 1981. In this hospital the post-natal wards were said to be operating a patient allocation system which meant that each mother came under

Table 4.2 *Distribution of social class of the sample by hospital*

	Social Class								
	1 and 2		3 n/m[a]		3 m[b]		4 and 5		Unclassified
	n	%	n	%	n	%	n	%	n	%
Hospital 1	40	52.1	19	48.7	26	38.1	21	24.0	6	54.5
Hospital 2	22	23.5	19	48.7	28	41.2	31	40.0	3	27.3
Hospital 3	23	24.3	1	2.6	14	20.6	22	36.0	2	18.2
Total[c]	85	30.7	39	14.1	68	24.5	74	26.7	11	4.0

[a] n/m, non-manual.
[b] m, manual.
[c] Two missing cases.

the care of a particular midwife. There was, however, no contact between this midwife and the mother before the baby was born, and observation of the ward during the study did not find that there was any real allocation of mothers to midwives. This was mainly due to the prolonged sickness of the sister normally in charge of the ward. Because of the number of other health districts from which this hospital drew its patients, there was no consistent policy of visiting by community midwives.

Research design

It would be unrealistic to study the relationship between mothers and midwives in isolation from the many other factors which have been shown to affect post-natal emotional well-being. Accordingly, the research design was based upon the concepts of the coping process and support systems. A number of factors arising from previous research were incorporated in the design in the hope of reducing possible distortion of the results by the presence of potent but unrecognised factors, and in order to compare any results related to midwifery care with those of other studies.

Factors in the research design

The factors included in the design were:

Personality of the mother (Pitt 1968; Kumar and Robson 1978; Wilson-Barnett 1979). This was assessed by the use of the Eysenck Personality Inventory, which provides a measure of anxiety trait and extroversion/introversion.

Maternal separation from her own mother before the age of 11 years (Frommer and O'Shea 1973; Brown and Harris 1978)

Life-crisis events occurring during the year preceding the birth (Holmes and Rahe 1967; Nuckalls, Cassell and Kaplan 1972; Kumar and Robson 1978). The life-crises included were:

death of a close family member
illness/injury of a close family member
changes in marriage/partnership
changes in residence or living conditions

changes in husband's employment
changes in own employment
any other stressful changes reported by the mother

Time of first holding the baby, time of first feeding the baby, any separation of mother and baby during the stay in hospital (Klaus and Kennell 1970, 1976, 1982).

Mother's reported feelings after the birth (Ball 1981).

Mother's self-image (Broussard and Hartner 1971; Lynch *et al.* 1976; Oakley 1980; Rosen and Stein 1980).

The research design is illustrated in Figure 4.1.

Working hypotheses

Two hypotheses were proposed:

The emotional response of women to the changes which follow the birth of a child will be affected by their personality and by the quality of the support they receive from family and social support systems.

The way in which care is provided by midwives during the post-natal period will influence the emotional response of women to the changes which follow the birth of a child.

Data collection from mothers

Data were collected form the mother on three occasions:

1. Each mother was recruited during a visit to the ante-natal clinic at around the thirty-sixth week of her pregnancy. During this interview a number of questions were asked about her personal circumstances, and about what she was most looking forward to or fearing concerning the impending birth. Most women said that they were most looking forward to 'getting it over with', but a number said they were most looking forward to being a mother. During this interview questions were asked about separation from the woman's own mother before the age of 11, and each woman was asked to complete the Eysenck Personality Inventory before she left the clinic.

2. Each mother was then visited in hospital within 24–36 hours after the birth of her baby. Before the interview a full record of the events of the labour and delivery was obtained. This interview took place in private at the mother's bed-side

Fig. 4.1. Model of research design for the study of the emotional needs of mothers during the perinatal and post-natal periods.

Conceptual bases: COPING PROCESS   SUPPORT SYSTEMS
                  (Lazarus 1966)   (Caplan 1969)

Antecedent factors (late pregnancy)

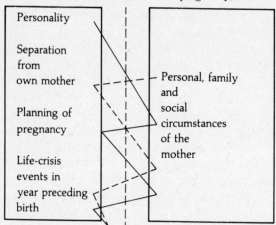

Personality

Separation from own mother

Planning of pregnancy

Life-crisis events in year preceding birth

Personal, family and social circumstances of the mother

Processes and events (birth and post-natal period)

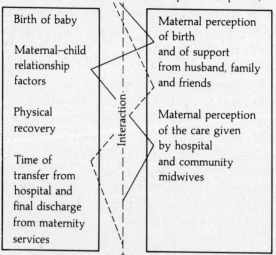

Birth of baby

Maternal–child relationship factors

Physical recovery

Time of transfer from hospital and final discharge from maternity services

Maternal perception of birth and of support from husband, family and friends

Maternal perception of the care given by hospital and community midwives

––Interaction·

Outcome (six weeks after the birth)

Measure of emotional well-being and satisfaction with motherhood. Mother's perception of current support from husband, family and friends

and allowed for the exploration of a number of issues. First the mother's perceptions of the birth were discussed and four rating scales were completed. These asked the mother to rank a number of questions about:

Her assessment of the birth as an experience in life as a whole

Her experience of labour and delivery compared with her expectation of it

Her perception of pain during labour

Her recall of her feelings immediately after the birth

With the exception of the pain perception scale, all the items were ranked from 1 to 5, with a further category for those women who felt that none of the statements offered adequately expressed her feelings. The pain perception scale was based upon Hayward's (1975) pain scale and the scores ranged from 'the pain was unbearable most of the time' to 'the pain never upset me during labour'.

During the rest of this interview the mother was asked about concurrent life-crisis events affecting her or her family, she was asked to recall the time when she first held and first fed her baby after delivery, and she was asked a number of other questions about the organisation of her post-natal care, and the amount of support she expected to receive from her family on her return home.

3. The mother was next contacted when the baby was six weeks old. At that time she was sent a postal questionnaire which was in three parts. Part 1 asked her to rate a number of items about her care in the hospital post-natal ward. Part 2 asked her to rate the care she had received from the community midwives. Part 3 was a questionnaire about her feelings about herself, the baby and the quality of support she was receiving at that time from her family. The structure of this questionnaire will be discussed more fully later.

Data collection from midwives

Data were obtained from midwives on two occasions:

1. On the day that each mother was sent home from hospital, the midwife responsible for arranging her transfer to the care of the community midwife was interviewed. During this interview the midwife was asked for her assessment of the physical and emotional state of the mother at the time of discharge, and

about her ability to cope with her baby. In a considerable number of cases the midwife arranging the transfer had not had much contact with the mother during the previous few days and made her judgements on the basis of the nursing records. These were also the basis of information sent to the community midwife about each mother.

2. Each community midwife received a questionnaire with an explanatory letter via the mother on her return home. The midwife was asked to complete the questionnaire on the day upon which the mother was finally discharged from the care of the domiciliary services. The community midwife was asked similar questions to those asked of the hospital midwife, and in addition was asked to record the time when the mother was first visited after her return from hospital, and the length of time after the birth during which the mother received care from the community midwifery services.

During the period of the study in each hospital non-participant observation of the post-natal ward was undertaken and notes kept of the way the wards were organised. The researcher also sat in at a number of shift report sessions, and examined the type of information sent to community midwives and health visitors.

Design, structure and factor analysis of the post-natal questionnaire

As previously stated, this questionnaire was in three parts. Parts 1 and 2 were concerned with the mother's perception of the care she received and her feelings during her stay in hospital and during the period when the community midwife was visiting her at home after delivery.

Hospital-based post-natal care

This questionnaire consisted of 16 statements designed to assess:
    Mother's self-image
    Her perception of infant feeding and the amount of help given
    Her ability to relax in the ward situation and the amount of rest she had
    Her perception of the support given by midwives

Post-natal care given at home

This questionnaire consisted of 14 statements designed to assess:
Mother's self-image
Her perception of her ability in feeding the baby
The amount of rest she had and the demands made by her family
Her perception of the support given by midwives

Scoring system

All the statements in the post-natal questionnaire were designed to allow a range of five responses, from 'strongly agree' to 'strongly disagree:'. These responses were scored from 1 to 5, with the score of 3 being given to a non-committal response of 'neither agree nor disagree' and the highest score to the most favourable response. For example, a positive statement such as 'I felt fit and well soon after my baby was born' would be scored as follows:

Strongly agree	Score 5
Agree	Score 4
Neither agree nor disagree	Score 3
Disagree	Score 2
Strongly disagree	Score 1

On the other hand, a negative statement such as 'I didn't feel well enough to look after my baby' was scored in the opposite direction, so that the most positive response again received the highest score, thus:

Strongly agree	Score 1
Agree	Score 2
Neither agree nor disagree	Score 3
Disagree	Score 4
Strongly disagree	Score 5

The statements were written in varied forms so as to avoid a response set (Oppenheim 1966). Two further questions were included. On the hospital-based questionnaire (part 1) the mother was also asked to indicate whether in retrospect she considered the time spent in hospital had been right for her or not. On the community-care-based questionnaire (part 2) mothers for whom it was appropriate were asked how their older child or children had reacted to the advent of the new baby. The answers to these questions were not included in the overall scores on the post-natal statements. In addition the mothers were invited to add any other comments they wished. The total score for parts 1 and 2 of the questionnaire was used in a limited way to assess mothers' overall reactions. The results of all the questionnaires were subjected to factor analysis and the factor scores which emerged from this process were then used as variables in the analysis. (Factor analysis is a statistical technique based upon intercorrelating all the items being investigated with each other, in order to abstract one or more underlying factors which the items have in common (Oppenheim 1966; Stopher and Meyburg 1979).)

Factor analysis

Six factors emerged from the hospital post-natal care questionnaire, and four from the questionnaire about post-natal care at home.

Hospital-based post-natal care

The formation of each factor emerging from the hospital-based questionnaire and the factor loading for each statement after Varimax rotation are listed below.

Factor 1. Feeding support factor
This was formed from the answers to four statements:

Statement	Factor loading
'The midwives and nurses were helpful when I was feeding my baby'	+ 0.83325
'I was helped to feel confident when I was feeding my baby'	+ 0.73999
'The midwives and nurses seemed to understand what help I needed'	+ 0.72584
'I needed more help in feeding my baby than I was given'	+ 0.54348

This factor was quite distinct from factor 5, which reflected the mother's perception of her own abilities and skill when feeding her baby during the early post-natal days in hospital.

Factor 2. Ward atmosphere
These four statements reflect anxiety which might be expressed by any patient in any hospital:

Statement	Factor loading
'I felt homesick and lonely'	+ 0.84173
'It was easy to relax and feel at home'	+ 0.57817
'I felt silly asking questions'	+ 0.56929
'Nobody listened to what I said, they just told me what to do'	+ 0.51631

Factor 3. Physical well-being
These statements formed this factor:

Statement	Factor loading
'I didn't feel well enough to look after my baby'	+ 0.85334
'I felt fit and well soon after my baby was born'	+ 0.82465
'Other mothers seemed to manage better than I did'	+ 0.46431

Factor 4. Rest
This proved to be a most interesting factor in the reactions of mothers to the different post-natal care practices in the different hospitals. It was formed from the following statements:

Statement	Factor loading
'It was easy to get enough rest in the day-time'	+ 0.83651
'I needed more rest at night'	+ 0.62377
'It was easy to relax and feel at home'	+ 0.59795

Factor 5. Self-image in feeding
This factor emerged consistently as quite separate from the feeding support factor. It was formed from the following statements:

Statement	Factor loading
'Feeding my baby was a worry'	+ 0.88433
'I needed more help in feeding my baby than I was given'	+ 0.58542
'Other mothers seemed to manage better than I did'	+ 0.58158

Factor 6. Conflicting advice
This final factor was formed from the following statements:

Statement	Factor loading
'Conflicting advice from midwives was upsetting'	+ 0.83843
'Different midwives gave different advice'	+ 0.81843

Post-natal care at home
The factor analysis of the questionnaire about post-natal care at home produced four factors. The factor formation and the factor loading for each statement in the factor after Varimax rotation are given below:

Factor 1. Midwife support
This factor was concerned with the mother's reaction to the way the midwives cared for her:

Statement	Factor loading
'The midwife seemed to understand what help I needed'	+ 0.86127
'The midwife's visit was a great help'	+ 0.83750
'The midwife always seemed to be in a hurry'	+ 0.67615

Factor 2. Continuity of advice
This factor reflected not only the advice received from midwives and health visitors, but also that given by family and friends:

Statement	Factor loading
'Different midwives gave me different advice'	+ 0.76022
'The health visitor and midwife gave conflicting advice'	+ 0.65232
'There were too many different midwives visiting me'	+ 0.64678
'Too many people gave me advice'	+ 0.64188

Factor 3. Rest/family support
These statements formed this factor:

Statement	Factor loading
'The family expected me to do too much'	+ 0.83766
'After I came home it was difficult to get enough rest'	+ 0.75567
'My husband seemed to know what help I needed'	+ 0.63743

Factor 4. Self-confidence
This factor reflects Pitt's description of a mother's confidence in caring for her baby

Statement	Factor loading
'I felt I couldn't cope on my own'	+ 0.78537
'I felt confident in handling my baby'	+ 0.77457
'I needed more help in feeding my baby than I was given'	+ 0.53812

Design, structure and factor analysis of the emotional well-being and satisfaction with motherhood questionnaire

It must be emphasised that the questionnaire was designed to provide a measure of the mother's self-report of her feelings six weeks after the birth of her infant. It is not an assessment of clinical depression, but it was derived from methods used in other studies and patterned upon the Beck Depression Inventory (BDI).

The BDI (Beck *et al* 1961) has been found to have a high degree of reliability, and self-evaluation using this inventory produced results which were consistent with independent clinical examination. Dewi-Rees and Lutkin (1971) found the BDI to be a suitable tool for their general-practice-based assessment of depression in parents before and after the birth of a baby. Pitt (1968) designed a questionnaire to assess post-natal depression that covers much of the same ground. Kumar and Robson (1978) used the Standardised Psychiatric Interview (Goldberg *et al.* 1974). However, this is designed to be used by psychiatrists trained in its methods, which made it unsuitable for use in the present study.

It was decided to base the questionnaire on the BDI and Pitt's questionnaire. It was not considered realistic to measure emotional well-being in isolation, and statements assessing the mother's satisfaction with motherhood and with the support she was receiving from her family were also included.

Certain items in the BDI were not included, either because they were considered inappropriate or because the same item was dealt with more appropriately in Pitt's questionnaire. For example, statements in the BDI based upon pessimism or self-punitive wishes including thoughts of death or suicide were thought to be potentially harmful in a questionnaire whose purpose was to explore the feelings of normal mothers.

Assessment of emotional well-being

A total of 19 statements were used to assess emotional well-being, based on Beck *et al.* (1961) and Pitt (1968).

Depression (Pitt)   Mood (Beck)   Crying spells (Beck)
  'Most of the time I feel happy and cheerful'
  'I've felt in low spirits since my baby was born'

Dependency (Pitt)   Sense of failure (Beck)
  'I feel confident about the way I cope'
  'I don't like to be left alone'

Anxiety (Pitt): (a) General, (b) Baby
  'I worry a lot'

Depersonalisation (Pitt): (a) Self, (b) Baby
  'Sometimes I feel I am a machine, not a person'
  'Sometimes it feels as if the baby doesn't belong to me'

Sleep disturbances (Beck, Pitt)
  'I sleep well when the baby will let me'

Irritability (Beck, Pitt)
  'I easily get upset if things go wrong'
  'I lose my temper more than I used to'

Guilt (Beck, Pitt) Self-hate (Beck)
  'I blame myself for problems with the baby'
  'If I had more help I would manage better than I do'

Indecisiveness (Beck)
  'I find it hard to make up my mind'

Appetite (Beck, Pitt)
  'I don't enjoy food the way I used to'

Libido (Beck, Pitt)
  'Sex doesn't interest me as much as before'

Work inhibition (Beck) Retardation (Pitt)
  'I feel full of energy these days'
  'I feel tired and weary'

Body image (Beck) Hypochondriasis (Pitt; also Gruis 1977)
  'Getting my figure back is important to me'

Assessment of satisfaction with motherhood

The statements about the role of mothering and the mother's perception of her infant's response were designed to assess her feelings about the responsibilities of mothering. The statements used were:
  'The time I spend with my baby is the best part of the day'
  'I talk to my baby quite a lot'
  'I feel that my baby knows that I love him/her'
  'Being a mother is satisfying'
  'Sometimes I wish I could go away on my own'
  'Caring for a small baby makes me feel nervous'
  'I enjoy stroking my baby's skin'
  A separate question which was not included in the total sum of scores on satisfaction with motherhood was added to assess further the mother's perception of her infant. This was patterned upon the Neonatal Perception Inventory devised by Broussard and Hartner (1971), and asked the mother to compare her infant with the 'average' baby in such areas as crying spells, feeding and sleeping patterns, and settling down into a routine. There

was no suggestion given in the inventory as to what 'average' was, as the criterion upon which it is based is the individual mother's perception of 'average' behaviour.

Assessment of quality of support

These statements were designed to assess the mother's perception of the availability and quality of help provided by family and friends, and her feelings about the amount of help she needed. Thus a statement such as:

'My family and friends are helpful'
would measure the degree to which she saw them as helpful, whereas a statement such as:

'Sometimes I feel overwhelmed by all that I have to do'
would measure how she felt about her situation irrespective of the help available to her.

The statements about the quality of family support are:

'I wish someone would tell me I'm doing a good job'
'My family and friends are helpful'
'Sometimes I feel overwhelmed by all that I have to do'
'My husband gives me all the help I need him to give'
'If I need help there is always someone I can turn to'
'Sometimes I feel lonely and isolated'

Factor analysis

The factor analysis produced seven factors from the 32 statements in the questionnaire. Five factors were centred upon emotional well-being, one on satisfaction with motherhood, and one on family support. The seven factors are listed below with details of their eigenvalues and factor loading:

	Eigenvalue	% of variance	Cumulative % of variance
Depression/mood factor	7.05457	22.0	22.0
Satisfaction with motherhood factor	2.64876	8.3	30.3
Coping ability factor	1.75662	5.5	35.8
Anxiety	1.58048	4.9	40.7
Family support factor	1.43080	4.5	45.2

| Sleep/anxiety | 1.26420 | 4.0 | 49.2 |
| Self-confidence | 1.14572 | 3.6 | 52.8 |

The factor formation and the factor loadings for each statement in the factor after Varimax rotation are given below:

Factor 1. Depression/mood

Statement	Factor loading
'I feel full of energy these days'	+ 0.71115
'Most of the time I feel happy and cheerful'	+ 0.64109
'I feel tired and weary'	+ 0.63796
'I've felt in low spirits since my baby was born'	+ 0.62998
'Sex doesn't interest me as much as before'	+ 0.50936
'I easily get upset if things go wrong'	+ 0.47312

Factor 2. Satisfaction with motherhood

Statement	Factor loading
'I feel that my baby knows that I love him/her'	+ 0.74798
'The time I spend with my baby is the best part of the day'	+ 0.65983
'Being a mother is satisfying'	+ 0.65878
'I talk to my baby quite a lot'	+ 0.63023
'I enjoy stroking my baby's skin'	+ 0.48598

Factor 3. Coping ability

Statement	Factor loading
'Sometimes I feel overwhelmed by all that I have to do'	+ 0.65084
'Sometimes I feel I am a machine not a person'	+ 0.61579
'If I had more help I would manage better than I do'	+ 0.58480
'Sometimes I wish I could go away on my own'	+ 0.50075

Factor 4. Anxiety

Statement	Factor loading
'I find it hard to make up my mind'	+ 0.72251
'I blame myself for problems with the baby'	+ 0.59533
'I easily get upset if things go wrong'	+ 0.54585
'I worry a lot'	+ 0.50554

Factor 5. Family support

Statement	Factor loading
'If I need help there is always someone I can turn to'	+ 0.80389
'My family and friends are helpful'	+ 0.76030
'Sometimes I feel lonely and isolated'	+ 0.39468
'My husband gives me all the help I need him to give'	+ 0.39269

Factor 6. Sleep/anxiety

Statement	Factor loading
'I sleep well when the baby will let me'	+ 0.61954
'Sometimes I feel as if the baby doesn't belong to me'	+ 0.58840
'Caring for a small baby makes me feel nervous'	+ 0.57560
'I feel confident about the way I cope'	+ 0.44552
'I don't like to be left alone'	+ 0.36831

This factor appears to be very like the description given by Pitt (1968) of the 'atypical' depression following childbirth. Pitt described the emotionally distressed women in his study as expressing anxiety about the baby and their ability to cope with the baby even though all the babies in his study were thriving.

Factor 7. Self-confidence

Statement	Factor loading
'I don't enjoy food the way I used to'	+ 0.74289
'I wish someone would tell me I'm doing a good job'	+ 0.54473

'Sex doesn't interest me as much as
before'   + 0.39929
'I lose my temper more than I used to'   + 0.37895

It can be seen that all the original statements derived from either Beck *et al.* or Pitt consistently loaded on to the emotional well-being factors (factors 1, 3, 4, 6 and 7). In addition, two statements designed to assess family support and two designed to assess satisfaction with motherhood also loaded on to the emotional well-being factors. These were the statements:

'I wish someone would tell me I'm doing a good job'
'Sometimes I feel overwhelmed by all I have to do'
'Sometimes I wish I could go away on my own'
'Caring for a small baby makes me feel nervous'

The use of the factor scores

A factor score for each factor was produced by adding together the scores for the mother's response to each of the statements which formed the factor. As was explained earlier, the response to each statement was scored from 1 to 5, and in each case the lowest score indicated the least favourable response. An example of a factor score is given below.

Example:Self-confidence factor (post-natal care at home)
This factor was formed from three statements:
'I felt confident in handling my baby'   score = 3
'I felt I couldn't cope on my own'   score = 2
'I needed more help in feeding my baby than I was given'
score = 4
        Total factor score = 9

The factors produced by the factor analyses were used as new variables in the analysis of the data, and two further variables were formed by adding together the scores given to all the statements in each part of the post-natal care questionnaire in order to produce a total score for hospital and domiciliary care.

*Emotional well-being/satisfaction with motherhood
and family support factor scores*

The emotional well-being questionnaire was designed to give an overall measure of the emotional state of the mother six weeks after the birth of her baby. Whilst it would have been interesting to compare different aspects of the factors for emotional well-being which were produced, it was decided to use the scores of the 23 statements which formed the five emotional well-being factors (factors 1, 3, 4, 6 and 7) to produce a total score which would provide a measure of the emotional well-being of the mother. Three of the emotional well-being statements appear more than once in the formation of the emotional well-being factors, but their scores were used only once in the combination of statement scores which made up the total emotional well-being score.

Extra information from the mothers

Each mother was invited to add further comments about any aspect of her post-natal care, or about her feelings at the time when she completed the post-natal questionnaire. This proved very useful as quite a number of the mothers used this facility to expand on some of their answers.

5

Some personal details about the mothers, their labour and delivery, and observations on post-natal care

Many of the mothers involved in the study said that they had enjoyed taking part and found it refreshing that their impressions and views of the midwifery service were being sought.

The outcome of the birth experience in terms of the mothers' emotional well-being will be discussed in the following chapters. This chapter will concentrate on the personal details of the mothers, the events of labour and the post-natal care the mothers received.

Personal details of the mothers

As described in the preceding chapter, 58.8% of the mothers were aged between 20 and 29 years, 35.4% were primigravidae and 42.3% were having their second child. One hundred and twenty-four mothers (44.4%) came from social classes 1, 2 and 3 non-manual, 142 (50.9%) from social classes 3 manual, 4 and 5, and the remaining 11 mothers were unclassified as regards social class. (No details were obtained for 2 mothers.)

Planning of the pregnancy

One hundred and eighty-eight mothers (67.4%) said that they had planned the pregnancy. There were no significant differences in the parity or social class of women who had planned the pregnancy and those who had not, but only 40% of women under 21 years of age had planned the pregnancy compared with 71% of those over 21 years. It had originally been decided to ask this question during the ante-natal interview, but many of the participants said they would prefer to discuss this matter after the baby was safely born, and it was therefore included in the post-labour interview. Some mothers said that they had a fear of 'ill wishing' the baby if they talked about its planning before it was born. It was found that whether the pregnancy was planned or not had no direct link with the subsequent emotional status of the mother.

Reported separation from own mother

A total of 33 women (12%) reported that they had been separated from their own mother for a period of at least three months before the age of 11 years. In most cases this was due to the death of the mother or the breakdown of the parents' marriage when the mother had relinquished the care of her daughter and had sporadic or no further contact. One woman included in this category said that she had been emotionally separated from her mother all her life!

Life-crisis events

A surprising number of women reported life-crisis events during the year of the pregnancy.

Sixty-one (22%) had suffered the death of a close family member, and one woman had been widowed during her pregnancy. She had nursed her husband until his death from Hodgkin's disease four months before their second child was born. Although she was still grieving the loss of her husband, she did not subsequently suffer from post-natal emotional distress.

Moving house or having major structural alterations to the house was frequently reported. Altogether 112 women (40%) moved house either during pregnancy or within six weeks of the infant's birth, or were still in the throes of major alterations at the time the baby was born.

Ninety women (32%) reported changes in their husband's employment during the pregnancy, 48 women (17%) were on maternity leave from their jobs, and a further 89 (32%) had given up a job entirely as a result of the pregnancy.

Thirty-seven women (13%) had either married or begun living with their male partners during the pregnancy.

During the post-labour interview each woman was asked whether there were any other events or situations apart from those listed above which had caused stress during the pregnancy. Fifty-two women (19%) reported marital or family tension, and 26 (9%) said that they were finding it very difficult to adjust to giving up work.

Labour and delivery

Categories of labour

Labour was classified into three categories:

1. *Spontaneous labour* was defined as one which began spontaneously and continued without any augmentation until completion. One hundred and twenty-three women (44.1%) had a spontaneous labour.
2. *Induced labour* was defined as labour which was artificially induced and then continued without further assistance or was augmented by intravenous Syntocinon until completion. Ninety-seven women (34.8%) had an induced labour.
3. *Active management of labour* fell into two sub-groups: delivery by caesarian section and labours that began spontaneously but were then augmented by intravenous Syntocinon. Fifty-eight women (20.8%) fell into the active management category, of whom 29 had a caesarian section and 29 an augmented labour ending in vaginal delivery. Of the caesarian sections 16 were elective and 13 were emergency procedures.

Delivery

One hundred and ninety-five women (70.1%) had a normal delivery, 50 (17.9%) a forceps delivery, 4 (1.4%) a breech delivery and 29 women (10.4%) a caesarian section. (No information was obtained for one woman.)

Length of labour and pain relief

The mean average length of labour was 7 hours, with 70% of the mothers having a labour of 8 hours or less. During labour 17 mothers did not use any form of pain relief and 36 did not have any sedation during the first stage but used nitrous oxide and oxygen (Entonox) for the second stage.

One hundred and forty-two mothers (51%) were given pethidine during labour and 66 (24%) had an epidural. A general anaesthetic was given to 16 women (6%) undergoing elective caesarian section.

Episiotomy

One hundred and thirty-two women (47%) had an episiotomy performed, 51 (18%) had a perineal tear, 7 (2%) had a perineal tear in addition to an episiotomy and 88 women (32%) had intact perinea.

Third stage

The third stage of labour was normal for 257 women (92.4%). Of the remaining 22 women, 12 had a post-partum haemorrhage, 9 had a retained placenta and 1 had a retained placenta which was accompanied by a post-partum haemorrhage. (Note: details of labour and delivery were missing for one case.)

Husband's presence

All the hospitals made it possible for the mother to have her husband or male partner or other helper of her choice with her during labour and delivery. In hospitals 1 and 3 this facility extended to the husband being present during caesarian section under epidural analgesia. In the event 184 women (66%) had a helper present throughout labour and delivery.

The babies

The sex distribution of the babies was even, with 140 boys and 140 girls being born. This number includes one set of undiagnosed twins (one boy and one girl) born to a 20-year-old primigravida.

All the babies were rated by the Apgar score at one minute after birth. Two hundred and twelve babies (76%) rated 8 or more at one minute; 9 babies (3%) were transferred to the special care baby unit after delivery. Most of these babies were returned to their mothers in the post-natal ward within 24 hours, and all of them were with their mothers by the fifth post-natal day.

Maternal contact with the baby after birth

All the hospitals had written policies which required that the baby be given to the mother to hold immediately after birth. When the mothers were asked about this event, 191 (68.5%)

said that they held their baby immediately after birth, and a further 51 (18.3%) said that although they did not hold their baby immediately they held him or her during the first hour after birth. Of the remaining 37 mothers, 16 (5.7%) held their babies within four hours, 9 (3.2%) within four to eight hours, and 12 (4.3%) did not hold their babies until more than eight hours had elapsed. Most of these incidences were due to the administration of a general anaesthetic.

One hundred and thirteen women (40.5%) fed their babies within the first hour after delivery and of these 85% chose to breast feed. It should be noted, however, that this figure represents only 58% of all the women who had chosen breast feeding as their method of feeding.

The mother's perception of labour and the birth of the baby

The scores given on the four rating scales designed to record the mother's perception of her labour and the birth produced some interesting results in view of the arguments which have raged in recent years about the management of birth in hospital.

Each mother was visited in the post-natal ward within 24–36 hours of the birth of her baby. The interviewer had familiarised herself with the details of labour and delivery contained in the obstetric records and after greeting the mother and admiring the baby, the interview usually began with the remark 'Well, what was labour like?' This led to a discussion during which the rating scales were completed.

Care received during labour

Almost without exception the mothers were full of praise for the care they had received during labour, and two particular facets of care emerged as having been most helpful.

The first was that one particular midwife, student midwife or in some cases medical student had been personally responsible for the mother's care throughout labour and the delivery, and it was frequently remarked that this had involved that person in staying with the mother after their shift had finished in order to complete the delivery. The mother, her husband and the midwife had used first names, and the picture which emerged was that where the mother felt a personal commitment to her and to her needs by the midwife or student, this had created a strong feeling of security and satisfaction.

These reports closely resemble those described in Shields' (1978) study of nursing care and labour and patients' maternal satisfaction. Shields interviewed 80 mothers following delivery; each described the care she had received and rated her level of satisfaction with particular aspects of that care. Mothers described the most helpful aspect of care as the nurse's sensitivity to their needs – nurses whose activity and attention in the labour ward were centred upon the mother and her partner and not 'just present in the room'. This sensitivity and attention was rated more highly than the degree of professional competence which the nurse had displayed.

The other aspect of care which drew favourable remarks was that in each of the three hospitals the mother had been carefully consulted about the use of drugs in labour and about any procedure which had been necessary. This approach to joint decision-making had been appreciated by most of the mothers, though some said that they felt the doctor or midwife should have made the decision. This latter group of women felt that they did not want the responsibility of making the decision and were happy to give it to their attendants. Others, however, felt just as strongly that this approach gave them the control they desired to have over their own labour.

The over-riding impression was that the quality of the relationship between the mother and her attendants led to a high degree of mutual respect and trust. Perhaps this is one of the reasons why the results of the labour perception rating scales do not substantiate the claims of certain pressure groups that any interference in the natural progression of labour inevitably produces dissatisfaction with the experience of birth. The results do underline, though, the strongly expressed need for each woman to be treated as a valued individual and to be involved in the decision-making process. They also indicate that some women prefer to give the responsibility for decisions to their attendants; that opinion also should be recognised and valued.

The rating scale results

All the mothers completed these scales even though those who had had an elective caesarian section had not experienced labour. These women often remarked that their 'labour pains' came after the birth, and related their answers to the way they felt on the first day after delivery. On each of the questions there were some mothers who felt that they could not express their feelings fully and that none of the responses adequately reflected how they felt. These 'no answer given' responses were allocated to a score of 3 which reflected the middle of the range of possible scores.

The results are given below:

Birth as a life experience
4 mothers (1.4%) said that the birth was the worst experience of their life
15 mothers (5.4%) said that it had been a bad experience
103 mothers (36.9%) said that it had been an important experience both good and bad
68 mothers (24.4%) said that it had been a good experience
76 mothers (27.2%) said it had been the best experience of their life
13 mothers (4.7%) did not answer

Mothers' experience of labour and delivery compared with their expectations of it
26 mothers (9.3%) said that the experience had been much better than they had expected
84 mothers (30.1%) said that it had been better than expected
61 mothers (21.9%) said that it had been as they had expected it would be
49 mothers (17.6%) said that the experience was worse than they had expected
30 mothers (13.9%) said that it had been much worse than they had expected
20 mothers (7.2%) did not answer

Mothers' reported feelings immediately after the baby was born
71 mothers (25.4%) said that they were gloriously happy
83 mothers (29.7%) said that they felt tired but happy
82 mothers (29.4%) said that they felt relieved
19 mothers (6.8%) said that they felt too tired to care

6 mothers (2.2%) said that they felt disappointed, and this was mainly due to the sex of the baby
18 mothers (6.5%) did not answer

The mothers' scores shown above were not found to be significantly related to age, parity or social class, nor to the type of labour and delivery.

The statistical details of these results and those which follow will be found in Tables 5.1, 5.2 and 5.3.

Mothers who fed their babies within the first hour after delivery rated the birth experience more highly than did those who did not feed their babies, and they also rated their feelings after the birth more highly than other mothers. This raises the question 'Which is the chicken and which is the egg?' Was the mother's remembrance of the birth richer because she had fed her baby, or did she feed her baby because she felt happy? Later analysis revealed that whether a mother fed her baby or not was related closely to her choice of feeding methods, her age and her parity and not to the type of labour or delivery, nor to whether she needed perineal suturing after delivery. These results will be discussed more fully later in relation to the mother's satisfaction with motherhood when the baby was six weeks old.

Pain scores
Perhaps it is not surprising to find that the mother's retrospective perception of pain in labour was closely related to the pattern of relief she had used, her parity, and to the length of the labour.

Primigravid women scored significantly lower scores (i.e. more pain experienced) than did multiparae ($P = 0.002$), and parity is also reflected in the scores of those who had a longer labour ($P = 0.04$) and those who had a forceps delivery ($P = 0.01$) (see Table 5.4).

The highest scores (i.e. indicating those who had not been upset by pain in labour) were those of 16 mothers who used no means of pain relief, and the next highest were those of the 40 women who had an elective epidural, closely followed by those who used only Entonox during the final stages of their labour. The 138 women who received pethidine during labour scored significantly lower scores, and the lowest of all came

Table 5.1 *Mothers' scores on labour perception scales classified by age and social class (Kruskall–Wallis one-way analysis of variance corrected for ties)*

Variable	n	Birth experience (mean rank score)	Expectation of labour (mean rank score)	Feelings after delivery (mean rank score)
(a) *Age of mother*				
17–20 years	31	143.8	141.9	153.0
21–29 years	161	139.0	138.4	130.8
30–39 years	84	135.6	137.5	147.8
		$\chi^2 = 0.2797, P = 0.8695$	$\chi^2 = 0.0724, P = 0.9664$	$\chi^2 = 3.9226, P = 0.1409$
(b) *Social Class*				
1	15	169.3	151.5	156.3
2	70	139.3	141.4	139.0
3 non-manual	38	163.3	145.0	141.8
3 manual	67	126.6	135.4	133.8
4	51	129.3	128.3	137.9
5	22	121.3	111.7	111.3
Unclassified	11	121.3	166.4	160.5
		$\chi^2 = 10.2568, P = 0.1142$	$\chi^2 = 5.0993, P = 0.5311$	$\chi^2 = 4.7913, P = 0.5708$

Table 5.2 Mothers' scores on labour perception scales classified by type of labour and delivery (Kruskall–Wallis one-way analysis of variance corrected for ties)

Variable	n	Birth experience (mean rank score)	Expectation of labour (mean rank score)	Feelings after delivery (mean rank score)
(a) Type of labour				
Spontaneous	121	137.5	146.7	131.6
Induced	97	139.0	123.3	148.4
Active Management	58	139.7	146.8	136.3
		$\chi^2 = 0.0409, P = 0.9798$	$\chi^2 = 5.6700, P = 0.0587$	$\chi^2 = 2.6064, P = 0.2717$
(b) Type of delivery				
Normal	194	142.5	142.5	137.7
Forceps	49	126.2	114.1	133.1
Breech	4	192.5	158.6	161.8
Caesarian section	29	121.6	150.0	149.8
		$\chi^2 = 4.8643, P = 0.1820$	$\chi^2 = 6.2598, P = 0.0990$	$\chi^2 = 1.2556, P = 0.7397$

Table 5.3 Mothers' scores on labour perception scales classified by parity and whether the baby was fed in the first hour after birth (Mann–Whitney U test corrected for ties)

Variable	n	Birth experience (mean rank score)	Expectation of labour (mean rank score)	Feelings after delivery (mean rank score)
(a) *Parity*				
Primigravidae	96	135.2	138.8	141.8
Multiparae	179	138.7	136.8	135.2
		$Z = -0.3654, P = 0.7148$	$Z = 0.2089, P = 0.8345$	$Z = 0.6870, P = 0.4921$
(b) *Feeding of baby in first hour*				
Fed baby	112	155.2	148.0	151.3
Did not feed baby	164	127.1	132.0	129.8
		$Z = 3.0193, P = 0.0025$	$Z = 1.6822, P = 0.0925$	$Z = 2.2760, P = 0.0228$

from those who had been given an emergency epidural after first having pethidine ($P = 0.0001$).

It should be noted that this was not a controlled trial and that many other factors which would have affected the perception and degree of pain were not recorded. The details of these results can be seen in Table 5.5.

Mothers' opinions about home versus hospital delivery

After all the details of the labour had been discussed, each mother was asked whether, in the light of the events of labour and delivery, she would have preferred the baby to have been born at home. A total of 28 mothers (10.1%) said that they would have preferred a home delivery.

Post-natal care in hospital

The organisation of post-natal care in hospital

The observed organisation of the post-natal wards was remark-ably similar in all three maternity hospitals. All the wards oper-

Table 5.4 *Mothers' scores on pain in labour scale classified by parity, length of labour and type of delivery*

	Variable	Pain perception	
		n	Mean rank score
(a)	*Parity*		
	Primigravidae	94	115.3
	Multiparae	174	144.9
	Mann–Whitney U test:	$z = -3.0202, P = 0.0025$	
(b)	*Length of labour*		
	4 hours or less	73	134.5
	5–8 hours	105	132.1
	9–13 hours	55	115.7
	13–20 hours	18	87.4
	Kruskall–Wallis test:	$\chi^2 = 8.1117, P = 0.0438$	
(c)	*Type of delivery*		
	Normal	194	137.2
	Forceps	48	110.1
	Breech	4	189.0
	Caesarian section	24	164.1
	Kruskall–Wallis test:	$\chi^2 = 10.5174, P = 0.0146$	

ated on a routine, task-based pattern of care which was mainly determined by the expected time that each mother would spend in the hospital after the birth of her baby.

The progress of care and helping the mother to gain skill and confidence in caring for her baby was arranged on a chronological basis. Mothers who had planned to go home within three days of the birth were not usually shown how to bath their babies whilst in hospital, but it was expected that this would be undertaken by the community midwife.

Supervision of infant care

In each hospital there was a routine pattern of care. On the first day of the baby's life the mothers were shown how to carry out a nappy change, clean the baby's bottom and wash his or her face. She was then expected to undertake this care for her baby from then on. On the second day mothers washed their babies, changed nappies and cot linen and fed their babies on demand, with the nursing staff giving support when asked. If the mother was not going home on the third day after delivery she undertook the daily bathing of her baby after a member of staff had demonstrated the correct technique to her. This regime did not appear to make any allowance for the age, parity or physical condition of the mother, who was expected to undertake a chronological progression of feeding and infant care.

Table 5.5 *Mothers' scores on the pain in labour scale classified by method of pain relief used*

Method of pain relief	Pain perception	
	n	Mean rank score
Epidural only	40	148.5
Epidural + sedation	24	91.1
Sedation ± Entonox	138	125.8
Entonox only	36	140.6
No pain relief	16	209.2
General anaesthetic[a]	14	154.0

Kruskall–Wallis test:
$\chi^2 = 27.1805$, $P = 0.0001$

[a] Applied to pain following anaesthetic.

One of the results of this routine approach was that mothers who had a painful perineum bathed their babies on the third post-natal day even though sitting on a chair was uncomfortable. For the same reason pain from the perineum was also a problem for mothers who were breast feeding.

The daily toilet care of the babies took place during the morning period and was mainly supervised by nursing auxiliaries, nursery nurses or junior student midwives. The supervision was allocated to staff on a task allocation basis. Thus a nursery nurse or student midwife might be told to 'see to all the baby baths'. The midwives concentrated on the physical assessment of the mother and discussion with her of the baby's feeding progress. It was not unusual to see a midwife carrying out her daily examination of the mother whilst the baby was being bathed in the nursery.

Division of care

Doctors tended to visit the wards most frequently during the morning shift and this diverted the midwife from the care of the mothers. Doctors also divided the care of the mother and baby, with obstetric housemen concerning themselves mainly with the physical care of the mother, and the paediatric housemen focusing on the care and well-being of the baby.

This fragmentation of care was reflected in the nursing records and reports. Although the nursery nurse or student midwife had supervised the care of the baby and recorded it in the notes she did not normally contribute to any report about the mother's level of skill or confidence in caring for the baby.

Hospital 3 had been included in the study because it claimed to be operating patient-centred care, but the pattern observed was for the mothers in each 'half' of the ward to be allocated to a particular midwife or student midwife for the morning shift. On the following day, although the same staff might be on duty, the allocation did not follow the same pattern but was likely to change according to the attitude of the midwife in charge of the wards. The allocation of staff to patients which had operated on one day did not form a basis for the allocation next morning.

The layout of the ward also affected the pattern of care. In hospital 2, which had Nightingale-type wards, there were very few occasions when nursing staff were not present in the wards, carrying out various tasks or talking to the mothers. In the other two hospitals, which had four-bedded rooms grouped around a central nurses' station, there were considerable periods of time when no nursing staff were to be seen in any of the four-bedded rooms. They tended to go into a room in order to carry out a particular task and then to group themselves in the office, at the central nurses' station, or in the nursery. This meant that there was much less natural interaction between mothers and nursing staff, and mothers were the main initiators of contact with midwives. This was particularly marked in hospital 3 because of the single corridor arrangement of the ward. The lack of windows in the corridor walls of the four-bedded rooms of hospital 3 made it difficult for the mothers to see staff moving from one room to another along the intervening corridor.

Supervision of infant feeding

The mothers were supervised when breast feeding on the first day after delivery. After the first day supervision was given as required and mothers were expected to feed their babies on demand, filling in a record of the feeds on a chart which was checked from time to time by the nursing staff.

Observation of this system revealed very few occasions when the midwife checked that the length of time the mother said that the infant had been breast fed really corresponded to the amount of time the child had sucked at the breast. Mothers were given advice and encouragement by midwives, but their approach to the feeding of their infants was not normally supervised after the first or second day unless they had been noted as having some difficulty. The advice given to mothers was varied and hardly ever recorded in detail in the nursing record. Instead, terms such as 'needs support' were used with no indication of the type of help needed or offered. Similarly, terms such as 'feeding well' were used to indicate babies of mothers who were seen as needing little or no further supervision. Breast feeding primiparae received more support in feeding than multiparous women, but primiparae who were bottle feeding were not given any more supervision than other mothers.

Mothers who bottle fed their babies were not usually supervised, but instructed to feed their babies at least every four hours and write the amount of feed taken on the feeding chart. Very little advice as to the amount of feed required was given. In the main bottle feeding mothers were given particular advice or supervision only when the baby was considered to be taking too little food, or when vomiting had occurred.

The research sample included 7 mothers who could not read or write competently. These women overcame the problems of the feeding chart by asking other mothers, or on a number of occasions the author, to fill in the chart on their behalf. At the time when these mothers were discharged from the hospital the midwife arranging for their discharge was asked whether she had realised that the mother could not read or write. With the exception of one mother, who was a gipsy and well known to the staff, the midwives had not been aware of the mothers' difficulties. Each of these women was bottle feeding, 4 were primigravidae, and all had been given written instructions about how to mix the baby's feed, about post-natal exercises, and about post-natal follow-up visits!

Pattern of infant feeding

At the time when the mothers were transferred from hospital post-natal care to either their own homes or to a GP maternity unit the pattern of infant feeding was as follows:

Breast feeding	161 mothers (57.7%)
Bottle feeding	93 mothers (33.3%)
Breast feeding + complementary bottle feeds	19 mothers (6.8%)
Missing information	6 mothers (2.2%)

At the time when the mothers were discharged from the care of the community midwife the feeding pattern was as follows:

Breast feeding	113 mothers (40.5%)
Bottle feeding	108 mothers (38.7%)
Breast feeding + complementary bottle feeds	14 mothers (5.0%)
Missing information*	44 mothers (15.8%)

*Because of the amount of missing information it is not possible to draw conclusions about the success or failure of breast feeding.

Fifty-four mothers (19.3%) were noted by the hospital midwives to be distressed and anxious about the feeding of their babies. Of these mothers 32 were breast feeding and 22 were bottle feeding. Observations of the ward patterns and discussions with the ward sisters did not reveal any system of assessing or planning post-natal care on an individual basis (apart from the decision about the length of time that the mother was likely to spend on the post-natal ward) except when some particular problem had been identified.

Rooming-in patterns

The policies for the rooming-in of mothers and babies in hospitals 1 and 3 were the same. Mothers had their babies by their bedside throughout the day and night from the second night after delivery. In some cases it was noted from observation and mothers' comments that the babies were left with their mothers at night from the day of delivery. The members of the night staff were discouraged from removing babies from their mothers' bedsides at night.

In hospital 2 the pattern was different, and the reason given was the cramped space available in the Nightingale-type wards. In this hospital the babies were taken to the nursery at night and brought to the mothers for feeding during the first two nights after delivery and thereafter according to the mothers' wishes. Most of the mothers went home on the third day after delivery and it was found that those who stayed longer mainly preferred their babies to go into the nursery at night.

Midwives' perceptions of the mothers during post-natal care in hospital

Physical well-being
The hospital midwives reported that 218 mothers (78.1%) had made a good physical recovery at the time they were transferred home. In view of the very short time which elapsed between the birth of the baby and the transfer home, this was taken to mean that the physical recovery of the mother from the trauma of the birth was progressing normally.

The assessment of physical recovery also tended to have its own ritual. In all three hospitals the midwife's arrangements for transfer home had to be endorsed by a physical examination of the mother by a junior hospital doctor. This usually took the form of fundal palpation and an examination of the perineum, with little or no reference to the baby's progress or the mother's wishes about her transfer home. This 'medical' approach tended to reinforce the attitude in some families that transfer from hospital meant that physical recovery was complete and that the mother could therefore assume her family responsibilities. It was not uncommon for a junior doctor to pronounce the mother fit for discharge only to find that the midwife had a good reason to recommend a longer stay in hospital (to enable the mother to rest or to acquire more confidence in caring for her baby, or because the community midwife had recommended it). In such cases it was often possible to come to a mutually satisfactory arrangement between the mother and the midwife, but there were also times of conflict and distress caused by such an approach which suggested that the only criterion for discharge was physical.

Emotional needs

During the interview of the hospital midwives, a number of questions were asked about the midwife's perception of the emotional status of each individual mother. The midwives described 218 mothers (78.1%) as appearing 'very happy' or 'placid' during their stay in hospital, 30 (10.8%) as showing a 'mixture of moods', 10 (3.6%) as 'withdrawn' and 7 (2.5%) as 'distressed'. No opinion was given for 14 mothers (5.0%). When asked in a further question whether the mother had suffered from the 'third day blues' or any other form of emotional distress only 3 mothers were considered to have had 'the blues' whilst 40 were said to have been distressed for other reasons, the main one of which was physical discomfort.

These reports are surprising in view of the fact that during a separate part of the interview the midwives were asked about certain symptoms of emotional distress which had been seen to affect the mothers during their stay in hospital. In answering this question the midwives cited 60 mothers as having wept during their stay, 41 mothers as having some degree of sleep disturbance, 37 to have shown signs of undue fatigue, 8 to have had a poor appetite, and 11 to have shown irritability!

It would appear that the midwives thought that some degree of emotional distress was 'normal' for post-natal women and did not consider this conflicted with their earlier assessment that 78.1% were 'happy' or 'placid'. This is borne out by the comments received from one mother who said 'all the midwives I have talked to say that this survey is a waste of time because all mothers get depressed and there's nothing to be done about it!'

This assumption meant that very little attention was paid to the emotional state of the mother when the arrangements for transfer home were made. It also meant that symptoms of emotional distress were not communicated to the community midwife.

The midwives seemed to be more sensitive to the feelings of mothers when the distress related to difficulties with feeding the baby. Fifty-four mothers (19.4%) were seen to be distressed about the feeding of their babies. Of these 30 were breast feeding and 24 were bottle feeding. A high proportion of the breast feeding women who were reported as being distressed changed from breast to bottle feeding in the hospital.

Later analysis did not reveal any significant difference in the age, parity or social class of the mothers who were reported as showing symptoms of emotional distress, the 'third day blues', or distress in feeding.

Transfer home and post-natal care in the community

Planned transfer home?

All the hospitals had a policy whereby the community midwife was asked to visit the mother at home during pregnancy and assess the length of time she was likely to need to spend in the hospital after delivery. The criteria for assessment were usually the condition of the mother's home and the amount of help she might expect from her family. The assessment was then recorded in the mother's obstetric notes and used as a basis for planning the length of post-natal care in hospital. It was rare to see the length of stay in hospital discussed with the mother after the birth of her baby, and decisions made during pregnancy did not appear to be changed in the light of the events of labour or delivery, or when the mother's home circumstances had changed since the assessment had been done.

Hospital 1 had a policy for the community midwife to visit the mother on three occasions during pregnancy and to make the final assessment approximately four weeks before the expected date of confinement.

During the period of the study in hospital 2 an area of disagreement arose between the hospital and community services and the policy of ante-natal assessment at home was not being followed. The community midwives were either not sending in a recommendation at all, or were assessing the mother's needs without visiting her home.

In hospital 3 there was a policy for mothers' needs to be assessed by the community midwife and for her to recommend the time of transfer home.

The effectiveness of the policies can be seen in Table 5.6, which shows that although 95% of the mothers in hospital 1 had been visited by a community midwife, the percentage was much lower in the other two hospitals.

Although only 28 mothers in hospital 2 had been visited, the community midwives made an assessment of need in 78 cases, and in hospital 3 the midwives made an assessment in 48 cases.

It is notable that hospital 1, which had the highest percentage of mothers visited in the ante-natal period, also had the highest percentage of mothers in social classes 1 and 2.

In hospitals 1 and 3 it was said that mothers could exercise some degree of choice about the length of time they stayed in hospital after the birth of their babies, but in hospital 2 a more rigid policy was pursued with all primigravid mothers being expected to stay in hospital or a GP maternity unit for a minimum of seven days. When the mothers were asked 'Did you have a choice in the length of stay in the post-natal ward?', 129 (47% of the total sample) said that they thought they had a choice; the highest percentage of these mothers was in hospital 1 where they had been visited by a community midwife. This is probably due to the facility provided for the mother to discuss her needs fully with the community midwife and then to review her decision near to the expected date of delivery. The arrangements for transfer home were more flexible in hospital 3 than in the other two hospitals.

One mother's comments upon the difficulty of reaching and being held to a decision taken early in pregnancy reflects the frustration which can occur:

I feel it is very hard to know when you are only three or four months pregnant how long you will need to stay in hospital. I had 10 days in hospital with my first baby – bearing this in mind I asked for seven days. But this time I could cope much better and felt well enough to go home after 3 or 4 days. I soon found out, however, that 7 day bookings remain 7 day bookings!

Another difficulty created by the system of deciding the time of transfer early in pregnancy is that any change which requires the mother to stay longer than was planned causes considerable distress. This tended to happen most frequently when the planned discharge was delayed because the baby had developed jaundice.

However, in spite of these observations most mothers felt that the length of time spent in hospital had been satisfactory. When the mothers were asked to comment six weeks after the birth on the length of time that they had stayed in hospital 219 (78.5%) felt that their stay had been about the right length of time, 37 (13.3%) said it had been too long and 20 (7.2%) said it had been too short.

Arrangements for transfer home and community care

Two hundred and thirty-three mothers (83.5% of the total sample) were transferred home before the baby was a week old, and of these 167 (59.9%) were transferred on or before the third day after the baby's birth. Forty-nine of the 167 mothers (17.6% of the total sample) were transferred to a GP maternity unit

Table 5.6 *Difference between hospitals in ante-natal visiting by community midwives*[a]

Hospital	The midwife visited		The midwife did not visit	
	n	%	n	%
1	107	95.5	5	4.5
2	28	26.4	78	73.6
3	36	58.1	26	41.9
	$\chi^2 = 102.47593$, 2d.f.; $P = 0.0001$			

[a] As reported by mothers.

before going to the care of the community midwife. The mid-wives often expressed frustration at the rapid turnover of mothers and babies passing through the post-natal wards, and said that this prevented them from giving individualised care to their clients.

It was not uncommon for the midwife who was arranging for a mother to go home to have had little or no direct contact with her in the preceding days. In all three hospitals a system operated whereby the midwife in charge of the ward automat-ically took responsibility for arranging for mothers to go home, and this routine pattern continued even when the midwife in charge had been off duty for the period immediately before the day of discharge. These midwives then relied upon the written notes, and when possible they consulted with their colleagues who had some direct knowledge of each particular mother. The transfer system, however, tended to be very routine in its approach, relying mainly on the arrangements made with the community midwife during the ante-natal period. These arrangements were usually implemented without question unless the mother or baby were considered to be 'having prob-lems'. 'Problems' were usually defined as difficulty in feeding, or the baby having some degree of jaundice. Very rarely was the mother's level of confidence taken into consideration.

When the mother was tranferred to the care of the community midwife very little information about her progress in the feeding or care of her baby was included on the routine information

Table 5.7 *Differences between hospitals in the length of community care*

Time of discharge from care of community midwife	Hospital 1		Hospital 2		Hospital 3		Total sample	
	n	%	n	%	n	%	n	%
On 10th day	2	1.9	2	2.3	3	7.3	7	3.0
11–20 days	2	1.9	42	48.3	25	61.0	69	29.6
21–28 days	85	81.0	37	42.5	9	22.0	131	56.2
29–35 days	16	15.2	6	6.8	4	9.8	26	11.1
Total[a]	105	100.0	86	100.0	41	100.0	233	100.0
			$\chi^2 = 82.78174$, 8 d.f.; $P = 0.0001$					

[a] Missing cases = 46.

which was sent to the midwife concerned. Occasionally the hospital midwife would discuss a mother with the community midwife via the telephone, but this was usually done in cases where some problem had occurred to do with the time of transfer home or the amount of help the mother could expect on her return home. All the hospitals had a prepared form on which information was sent to the community midwife concerning the date of birth of the baby, details of the labour and delivery, blood samples taken from the mother and baby, and the type of feeding and time of transfer home. The standardised nature of these forms allowed very little opportunity to give further information.

The most usual person to care for the mother on her return home was her husband (40.0% of the sample), followed by her mother or mother-in-law (31.0%). A number of mothers (17.6%) were looked after by both husband and mother or mother-in-law, and the rest were cared for by other relatives or friends (9.2%) or by no one (2.2%).

Midwives' perception of the mothers during post-natal care at home

The community midwives visited 44% of the mothers on the same day that they were discharged from hospital, and a further 52.3% of the mothers were visited on the morning of the day after discharge from the hospital.

They described 54 mothers as showing signs of emotional distress after their transfer home from hospital, and of these 17 were said to have 'third day blues' while 37 had distress due to other circumstances such as physical discomfort or lack of sleep. The community midwives noted 49 mothers as being tearful, 74 as not having enough sleep, 33 as showing undue fatigue, 27 as having signs of irritability and 17 as having poor appetite. They also noted that lack of sleep and undue fatigue affected mothers in the 30+ age group more than any other, but apart from that distinction there were no differences in the age, parity or social class of mothers showing signs of emotional distress.

At the time of discharge from the community midwifery service the midwives considered that family support for the mother had been 'very good' for 67.9% of the mothers, and 'good' for a further 26.6%.

At the time of transfer from hospital 161 babies (59.0%) were totally breast fed, 93 (34.0%) totally bottle fed and 19 (7.0%) were being breast fed and receiving complementary bottle feeds as well. (No information available for 6 babies.) The community midwives reported that 31 mothers had changed their method of feeding after they arrived home. Unfortunately the community midwife report was not received for 44 mothers, and this prevents a detailed analysis of changes for individual mothers. However, at the time when the mothers were discharged from the care of the community midwife 113 (48.0% of those reported) were feeding their babies by breast only, 108 (46.0%) were bottle feeding, and 14 mothers (6.0%) were still giving breast feeds topped up with bottle feeds.

Continuity of care from one or two midwives was more usual in the community. The midwives reported that 59.9% of the mothers had been attended throughout their period of domiciliary care by only two different midwives, and 29% of the mothers were attended by three different midwives. Seventy-six per cent of the mothers were visited by their health visitor during the time when the midwife was giving daily post-natal care.

The trend for midwives to visit mothers at home for longer than the statutory minimum of 10 days is shown in the report of the length of domiciliary care (Table 5.7). Only 7 mothers (3.0%) were discharged on the tenth day after the baby's birth, and 69 (29.6%) were discharged between 11 and 20 days after the birth. One hundred and thirty-one mothers (56.2%) were discharged between the twenty-first and twenty-eighth day after the birth. The remaining 26 mothers (11.2%) for whom data was obtained were discharged by the thirty-fifth day after the birth.

The pattern of post-natal care reported in this chapter is typical of that provided by the maternity services of the National Health Service at the present time. The majority of mothers are transferred to the care of the community midwife two or three days after the birth of the baby. The bulk of post-natal care therefore takes place in the community. Although the pattern of early transfer home has been typical of maternity care for a number of years, the continuation of community care beyond the tenth post-natal day is a comparatively recent development.

6

Factors surrounding the mothers' emotional well-being six weeks after the birth

Defining emotional well-being

The purpose of the study was to examine the effects which the post-natal support given to mothers by midwives might have upon maternal emotional well-being, and to consider the role played by midwives in the light of factors which had been found significant in other studies of post-natal emotional status and satisfaction. The measures of emotional well-being, satisfaction with motherhood and perception of post-natal care were obtained from the mothers' answers to the various statements which made up the post-natal questionnaire.

The factor analysis of the questionnaire, which is described in Chapter 4, indicated that the answers to 23 statements clustered together to form five emotional well-being factors. These factors were: depression, including loss of libido; coping ability; anxiety; sleep disturbance associated with anxiety; and self-confidence. The scores given on each of these factors were added together to form the emotional well-being (EWB) score. (For details of the scoring system used see p.51).

The results were as follows:

The range of possible EWB scores was from 23 to 115
The range of actual EWB scores was from 46 to 108
The mean average EWB score was 78.179
The standard deviation was 7.516

Although wherever possible the whole range of EWB scores was used in the analysis of the results, it was necessary to define low, moderate and high emotional well-being, both to assist certain methods of analysis and to compare the women classed as having low emotional well-being with those described by earlier research. In order to do so the following methods were used:

Women who had a total EWB score of 68 or less, which represents a mean average score of 2.95 or less per statement, were defined as the low emotional well-being group and considered to be emotionally distressed. There were 54 women in this group and they formed 19.4% of the total sample.

Women with low emotional well-being

The scores of the women who formed the low emotional well-being group revealed that they had symptoms similar to those of the depressed group described by Pitt (1968). They exhibited depression, anxiety and guilt (especially about the baby), sleep disturbance, tiredness, and lack of confidence in their ability to cope with the needs of the baby. All the babies were thriving at the time when the mothers completed the emotional well-being questionnaire.

There were other similarities between the emotionally distressed group in this study and those described by Pitt. He noted that the depressed women in his study had felt physically unwell in the early post-partum period, and that these feelings were quite distinct from those of the 'third day blues'. Their depression, which began in the hospital and grew worse when they first returned home with the baby, was experienced chiefly as tearfulness, feelings of inadequacy and inability to cope.

A similar picture was seen when a mother's score on the post-natal care questionnaire was examined in relation to her EWB score. Women whose scores for post-natal care in hospital indicated that they had not felt fit and well during their stay in hospital had significantly lower EWB scores, and a further significant relationship was found between their scores for self-confidence when they returned home with the baby and their EWB scores.

As mentioned above, the 54 women defined as emotionally distressed formed 19.4% of the total sample, which is a higher percentage than that found in earlier studies (Tod 1964; Pitt 1968; Dalton 1971; Kumar and Robson 1978). This can be accounted for by the difference between the definition of emotional distress used in this study and the firm clinical diagnosis of post-natal depression used in the other studies. However, although Pitt (1968) restricted his sample to those mothers with post-natal depression he also noted a further 19 women whom he classed as 'doubtfully depressed'. It is likely that many of the mothers classed as emotionally distressed in this study would have come into Pitt's category of doubtfully depressed, although some were considered to be depressed on the basis of their responses on the Beck Depression Inventory statements.

The similarities which exist between Pitt's description of mothers suffering from 'atypical depression', the criteria of depression included in the Beck Depression Inventory and the scoring patterns of the emotionally distressed group in this study suggest that the emotional well-being questionnaire was an effective tool in the differentiating between the different levels of emotional well-being expressed by the 279 women who formed the total sample.

It must also be recognised that the mother's feelings at the time of completing the questionnaire would have had a marked effect upon her responses, and care must be taken to distinguish between results which may be considered to be a further reflection of her emotional state at that time and those which indicate other factors and events which contributed to emotional outcome. The analysis of the results was therefore designed to assess the relationship which a variety of factors and events had with the different levels of maternal emotional well-being.

Analysing the results

In the analysis of results the whole range of EWB scores were compared with antecedent factors in the mothers, the events of the labour, delivery and post-natal care, and the scores given to post-natal care factors and satisfaction with motherhood. The statistical methods used included rank correlation and chi-square analysis, but the methods used most frequently were the Mann–Whitney U test (M–W) and the Kruskall–Wallis one-way analysis of variance by ranks (K–W). Both of these rank observations in order from the lowest to the highest and then determine whether the rank order of two or more different groups is so different that the groups are not likely to come from the same population. For example, the Mann–Whitney test was used to analyse the effect of parity on the rank order of the mother's score on the pain in labour scale. Primigravidae were put in group 1, multiparae in group 2. The results showed that most of the group 1 scores fell in the lower ranks while most of the group 2 scores were in the middle and higher ranks. The probability that the scores came from the same population was assessed as less than 0.01, indicating that the difference between the two groups was statistically significant and not due to underlying random error. The use of statistical methods reduces the danger that the researcher's own opinions on, for example, parity and the mechanisms of labour, would result in a biased judgement of the significance of the results based upon subjective feelings rather than well-grounded evidence.

Overview of the results

Three main parameters were identified, each of which contributed to the mother's emotional well-being but which arose from differing circumstances. For the sake of clarity it is necessary to discuss these parameters separately, but it must be remembered that they were part of a complex and dynamic interactive process in which some factors were seen to increase emotional conflict while others reduced it.

The three main parameters were:

1. Anxiety and its effects
There was a close relationship between anxiety and emotional outcome which also affected maternal perception of self-confidence and support.

2. Stress related to life-crises and post-natal care
The coping process was affected by additional stress arising from certain life-crisis events and particular aspects of post-natal care.

3. Satisfaction with motherhood
A relationship between emotional well-being and satisfaction with motherhood indicated that maternal satisfaction may increase emotional well-being but is itself affected by factors in the mother and in the management of her care.

These will all be discussed in detail below.

Factors which were not related to emotional outcome

The analysis also revealed that a number of major variables were not related to emotional well-being. These included the following:

The personality trait of extroversion/introversion measured by the Eysenck Personality Inventory approximately four weeks before the birth of the baby.

Maternal separation from her own mother before the age of 11 years.

The age and parity of the mother.

The type of labour and delivery experienced by the mother.

The time the mother spent in hospital.

The time for which the mother was visited by the community midwife.

The Eysenck Personality Inventory (EPI) is a trait test of extroversion/introversion and neuroticism/anxiety. (Eysenck and Eysenck 1968; Eysenck, Soueif and White 1969). The client's response to a series of questions produces two scores: the 'E' score, which gives a measure of extroversion/introversion, and the 'N' score, which is a measure of neuroticism/anxiety.

Extroversion/introversion

In the initial analysis of the results of individual hospitals, no significant relationship was found between the mothers' score on the extroversion/introversion scale on the EPI and her eventual EWB scores.

There were no significant differences in the distribution of either the extroversion/introversion scores or the anxiety/neuroticism scores of the mothers cared for by the three different hospitals, and the extroversion/introversion scores were eliminated from further analysis (Ball 1983[a]).

Separation

Although Frommer and O'Shea (1973) found that women separated from their mothers before the age of 11 years were more likely to have difficulty in adjusting to motherhood, no significant differences were found between the EWB scores of the 33 women in this study who reported such separation and the remainder of the sample who did not (M–W test; $P = 0.4664$). There was, however, a marked difference between the EPI anxiety/neuroticism (EPI(N)) scores of the separated women and the non-separated women (M–W test; $P = 0.0002$). This suggests that the separation had an effect upon the developing personality of the women concerned, adding weight to Brown and Harris's (1978) conclusion that separation is a predisposing factor in the incidence of depression among vulnerable women (see Table 6.1.)

Age and parity
There were no significant differences in the mothers' EWB scores as a result of age or parity.

Labour and delivery
Women who had an induced labour scored higher mean average EWB scores than those who had either a normal or actively managed labour, but the difference was not statistically significant (K–W test; $P = 0.2504$). (Women who had a caesarian section were included in the actively managed group.)

There were virtually no differences in the EWB scores of women who had a normal delivery, a forceps delivery or a caesarian section, but the four women who had a breech delivery scored very low EWB scores. A weak statistically significant difference was noted between the scores of the women in the breech group and those who had other forms of delivery, but this is distorted by the extremely small number concerned. It is concluded, therefore, that there was no significant relationship between emotional well-being and the form of labour or delivery the mother experienced. (Details of these results can be seen in Table 6.2.)

Table 6.1 *EPI(N) scores and EWB scores classified by separation/non-separation from own mother before the age of 11 years* (Mann–Whitney U test corrected for ties)

	EPI(N)		EWB	
	n	Mean rank score	n	Mean rank score
Separated from own mother	32	180.6	33	128.5
Not separated from own mother	233	126.4	242	139.3
	$z = 3.7714; P = 0.0002$		$z = -0.7283; P = 0.4664$	

Factors which were significantly related to post-natal emotional well-being

The three main factors which were found to be significantly related to post-natal emotional well-being were anxiety, stress associated with concurrent life-crisis events, and stress associated with certain aspects of post-natal care.

Anxiety and its wide-ranging effects

Although the personality trait of extroversion/introversion was not significantly associated with post-natal emotional well-being, that of anxiety/neuroticism was a powerful influence on the mother's reactions throughout the six weeks of the puerperium. Anxiety affected the mother's perception of her care in hospital and of the support she received from her family when she returned home. High levels of anxiety trait were associated with lower social class and bottle feeding.

Table 6.2 *EPI(N) scores and EWB scores classified by age, parity, type of labour and delivery*

	EPI(N)		EWB	
Variable	n	Mean rank score	n	Mean rank score
Age of mother				
17–20 years	30	146.7	31	146.4
21–30 years	155	140.4	164	135.3
31–39 years	83	119.1	84	146.8
K–W test:	$\chi^2 = 4.9598; P = 0.0838$		$\chi^2 = 1.3637; P = 0.5057$	
Parity				
Primigravidae	92	134.6	98	142.6
Multiparae	175	133.7	179	137.0
M–W test:	$z = 0.0995; P = 0.9208$		$z = 0.5485; P = 0.5833$	
Type of labour				
Spontaneous	116	131.8	123	133.0
Induced	94	130.6	97	150.4
Actively managed	57	144.1	58	135.0
K–W test:	$\chi^2 = 1.2468; P = 0.5361$		$\chi^2 = 2.7696; P = 0.2504$	
Type of delivery				
Normal	188	136.4	195	142.8
Forceps	47	132.3	50	132.2
Breech	4	99.5	4	34.0
Caesarian	28	125.9	29	144.3
K–W test:	$\chi^2 = 1.3156; P = 0.7254$		$\chi^2 = 7.7362; P = 0.0518$	

Anxiety and emotional well-being

A strong relationship was found between a mother's EWB score recorded six weeks after the baby was born and her level of anxiety measured by the anxiety/neuroticism (N) scale on the EPI approximately four weeks before the baby was born (K–W test; $P = 0.0001$).

As can be seen from Table 6.3, mothers in the low emotional well-being group had much higher EPI(N) scores than the rest of the sample. This link between anxiety/neuroticism and emotional well-being provided further confirmation of the similarity between the results of this study and those of Pitt's (1968) study. He found a significant relationship between post-natal depression and high anxiety/neuroticism scores measured on the Maudsley Medical Inventory (Eysenck 1959), which was the forerunner of the EPI (Eysenck and Eysenck 1968).

This result amply illustrates Lazarus's contention that anxiety is a powerful force in the coping process and that it may be present both as an antecedent factor in the form of a personality trait and as a contributory factor in the form of state anxiety aroused in response to stress (Lazarus 1966, 1969).

Kumar and Robson (1978) used the EPI to assess the relationship between personality and post-natal depression in a sample of 119 primigravidae. In their study the EPI was completed during the first trimester of pregnancy and the assessment of post-natal depression was undertaken three months post-delivery. Kumar and Robson did not find a significant relationship between high EPI(N) scores and post-natal depression. Although the difference in the timing of the two measures makes direct comparison difficult, their results suggest that any

Table 6.3 *EPI(N) scores compared with post-natal EWB scores* (Kruskall–Wallis one-way analysis of variance)

EWB	n	EPI(N) (mean rank score)
Low scores	54	186.4
Moderate scores	187	125.7
High scores	27	91.6
K–W test:	$\chi^2 = 35.0252; P = 0.0001$	

relationship between anxiety trait and emotional distress reduces with the passage of time. If this is so, then it is an indication that anxious women need a longer time than less anxious women to adapt to motherhood.

People with high anxiety trait as measured by the EPI are not highly neurotic, but can be described as timid, fearful, very sensitive to criticism and anxious to please. Women generally score higher than men, and working class people score higher than any other social class (Eysenck and Eysenck 1968; Eysenck *et al*. 1969).

Anxiety and social class

The link between anxiety and social class is another indication of the complexity of the situation surrounding vulnerability to depression (Brown and Harris 1978) and it emerged in the results of this study. The mothers in social classes 3 manual (m), 4 and 5 had higher EPI(N) scores than those in social classes 1, 2 and 3 non-manual (n/m) (M–W test; $P = 0.0003$). The mothers in social classes 3m, 4 and 5 also had lower EWB scores than the women in social classes 1, 2 and 3 n/m (M–W test; $P = 0.0038$). However, the degree of statistical significance of the correlation between social class and anxiety is higher than that between social class and emotional well-being, and this suggests that the link between social class and emotional well-being can be attributed to the underlying personality factor. The details of the relationship between social class, personality, emotional well-being and choice of infant feeding method are given in Table 6.4.

Anxiety and choice of feeding method

The close relationship between anxiety and social class described above was found to be a factor in the difference between the EWB scores of the mothers who breast fed their babies and those who bottle fed (see Table 6.4). Working class mothers are known to choose bottle feeding more often than breast feeding (Jackson, Wilke and Auerbeck 1956; Hytten, Yorkston and Thomson 1958; Bacon and Wylie 1976; Houston, 1981). In the present study 51.4% of the mothers in social classes 3m, 4 and 5 chose to bottle feed their babies compared with 12.5% of the mothers in social classes 1, 2 and 3 n/m. Mothers of all social

classes who bottle fed their babies had higher EPI(N) scores
before the baby was born (M–W test; $P = 0.0012$) and lower
EWB scores six weeks after delivery than the breast feeding
mothers (M–W test; $P = 0.0211$). Once again the degree of difference between anxiety and choice of feeding method is greater
than between emotional well-being and feeding method, indicating that the link between anxiety and social class is also a
factor in the choice of infant feeding method. If this is so then
it brings a new dimension into the approach which professional
staff should have towards encouraging women to breast feed
their babies. The anxious woman may choose to bottle feed in
order to avoid the effect which she perceives the difficulty of
breast feeding may have upon her fragile coping resources. Any
overt disapproval of her choice will cause guilt and distress and
is likely to undermine her confidence.

Anxiety and adjustment to motherhood
Another set of interactive relationships was found between a
mother's ante-natal EPI(N) scores, her feelings of physical and
emotional well-being in the post-natal ward, her self-confidence
and perception of support when she returned home and her
emotional well-being six weeks after delivery. The physical well-
being factor score indicated whether or not the mother had felt

Table 6.4 *EPI(N) scores and EWB scores classified by social class and
choice of infant feeding method*

Variable	EPI(N)		EWB	
	n	Mean rank score	n	Mean rank score
Social class[a]				
1 and 2	83	107.3	85	141.4
3n/m	38	118.1	39	162.7
3m	61	137.9	68	123.1
4	51	153.0	51	120.2
5	23	142.8	23	115.2
K–W test:	$\chi^2 = 15.0342; P = 0.0046$		$\chi^2 = 10.6218; P = 0.0312$	
Choice of feeding method				
Breast	156	119.0	161	146.2
Bottle	106	149.9	112	123.8
M–W test:	$z = -3.2431; P = 0.0012$		$z = 2.3068; P = 0.0211$	

[a] Eleven unclassified mothers not included.

fit and well during the time she spent in the post-natal ward. The ward-atmosphere factor score indicated her feelings about being in the hospital; whether she felt relaxed and at home, freely able to ask questions and obtain help, or whether she felt homesick and lonely, and afraid to ask questions.

The mothers who gave low scores on these factors had significantly higher EPI(N) scores than the rest of the sample, and they also had lower EWB scores (see Table 6.5). The anxious women found it less easy to relax and feel at home in the ward, and their anxiety was manifested in physical as well as emotional symptoms. There is no evidence to suggest that the anxious mothers received poorer care than the rest of the mothers in the same ward, but their natural anxiety made it more difficult for them to cope with the strange environment.

The study of medical patients provides further evidence of the difficulty which people with high anxiety trait have in adjusting to hospital. In a study by Wilson-Barnett and Carrigy (1978) the trait anxiety levels of non-urgent medical patients admitted to one ward were assessed on the (N) scale of the EPI on the day of their admission to hospital. The patients' state anxiety was then assessed daily by the Lishman Mood Adjective List (Lishman 1972) for as long as they remained in the hospital. The patients who had high EPI(N) scores on the day of admission manifested much higher levels of state anxiety than the other patients in the same ward, and their anxiety remained high for at least five days after admission.

Table 6.5 *EPI(N) scores and EWB scores compared with scores for post-natal ward atmosphere and physical well-being*

Variable	EPI(N)		EWB	
	n	Mean rank score	n	Mean rank score
Ward atmosphere	78	153.4	77	102.9
Moderate scores	115	130.6	125	146.4
High scores	75	120.8	77	155.5
K–W test:	$\chi^2 = 7.3102; P = 0.0259$		$\chi^2 = 15.7959; P = 0.0004$	
Physical well-being				
Low scores	44	156.5	46	95.7
Moderate/high scores	224	130.2	233	148.8
M–W test:	$z = 2.0624; P = 0.0392$		$z = -4.0802; P = 0.0001$	

Anxious people find it difficult to relax, to take in information and to learn new skills. It is not realistic, therefore, to expect anxious mothers to learn how to care for their babies and to cope with carrying out that care at the same pace as less anxious mothers. They will need more time to become confident and may need to have the same information imparted on a number of occasions before they make full use of it. Anxious people become more anxious when they feel that they are not conforming with others' expectations of them.

The interactive relationship between anxiety trait and emotional well-being is seen again in the mother's scores for self-confidence and perception of family support when she returned home with the baby (see Table 6.6). The mothers who scored low on these factors had higher EPI(N) scores and lower EWB scores than the other mothers.

The reports from the community midwives support the mother's retrospective rating of her confidence when she returned home with the baby. They recorded that 54 mothers had shown signs of emotional distress within a few days of their return from the hospital. Six weeks later these mothers rated their self-confidence in the early days at home as poor, and their scores were significantly lower than those of the rest of the sample (M–W test; $P = 0.0060$).

Mothers who rated the quality of their support from their families as low also had higher EPI(N) scores (M–W test;

Table 6.6 *EPI(N) scores and EWB scores compared with scores for self-confidence and family support at home* (Mann–Whitney *U* test corrected for ties)

		EPI(N)	EWB
Variable	n	Mean rank score	Mean rank score
Self-confidence at home			
Low scores	28	163.4	45.3
Moderate/high scores	240	131.1	146.5
M–W test:		$z = 2.0807; P = 0.0369$	$z = -5.1490; P = 0.0001$
Family support at home			
Low scores	76	156.9	90.3
Moderate/high scores	188	122.6	155.4
M–W test:		$z = 3.3079; P = 0.0009$	$z = -5.7278; P = 0.0001$

$P = 0.0009$) and lower EWB scores than any other group (M–W test; $P = 0.0001$) (see Table 6.7). This time the community midwives' assessment of the quality of the support the mother received from her family did not coincide with that of the mother, suggesting that it is not the amount of support which matters to the mother but the quality of that support in relation to her emotional needs and confidence.

There is no doubt that personality was a powerful influence upon the way women coped with the demands of motherhood, and that anxious women were more vulnerable to emotional distress.

Pitt's study (1968) found a similar pattern of physical and emotional distress, lack of confidence and dissatisfaction with family support among his depressed mothers. It is difficult to determine to what extent the low scores for physical and emotional well-being in the ward and lack of confidence and family support at home were due to the underlying effect of high anxiety and to what extent these feelings were signs of developing post-natal distress.

The high degree of significance between the scores for the post-natal care factors and the EWB scores suggests that many of the mothers who felt unwell and unhappy in hospital and

Table 6.7 *Mothers' scores for self-confidence, family support, emotional well-being and satisfaction with motherhood classified by midwives' observations of maternal emotional distress during the first week at home* (Mann–Whitney U test corrected for ties)

Factors	Midwives' observations	
	Emotional distress seen (mean rank scores; $n = 54$)	Emotional distress not seen (mean rank scores; $n = 183$)
Self-confidence	97.1	125.5
	$z = -2.7504; P = 0.0060$	
Family support	108.9	122.0
	$z = -1.2612; P = 0.2072$	
Emotional well-being	104.0	123.4
	$z = -1.8294; P = 0.0673$	
Satisfaction with motherhood	116.2	119.8
	$z = -0.3455; P = 0.7297$	

who lacked confidence at home were showing early signs of the emotional distress which was still present six weeks later.

Many mothers experience some degree of emotional disturbance in the early post-natal period, but this usually passes as confidence grows. For a number of vulnerable women, however, this distress did not pass away but signalled a spiralling situation of anxiety, lack of confidence and emotional distress.

Stressful life-events

The main focus of this study is the major life-event of pregnancy, childbirth and the mothering of a new infant. It would be foolish, however, to assume that this was the only major life-event being experienced by the mothers and their families, and many of the mothers in the sample reported other life-crises which had occurred during the year preceding the birth of the baby. These included the death or serious illness of a close family member, marriage or the separation of couples, changes in the mother's or her husband's employment, and either moving house or having major alterations done to the house. In addition, the mothers volunteered information about other stressful events. These fell into two main categories: marital and family conflict, and difficulty in adjusting to the loss of an interesting career.

Altogether 456 life-events were reported by the 279 mothers in the study. For many of them therefore, the birth of a baby was one more stressful event to cope with in an existing situation of adjustment and stress.

The relationship between life-events and emotional well-being is shown in Table 6.8. It can be seen that there were no significant differences in the EWB scores of women who reported the death or illness of a family member, marriage or separation, or changes in the husband's employment compared with women who did not suffer these stresses. But women who reported marital tension or a disturbance to the home, i.e. moving house or having major alterations done, scored significantly lower levels of emotional well-being. The degree of significance between the scores of the mothers who moved house and those who did not is not high; this life-event is included because it affected 112 mothers (40% of the sample) and because an association between moving house and severe post-natal depression has been observed in clinical practice (M. Oates, personal communication).

Marital conflict

A relationship between marital conflict and depression in women has been demonstrated in other studies of post-natal difficulties (Tod 1964; Nuckalls *et al.* 1972; Kumar and Robson 1978; Oakley 1980), and in a study of the role of social factors in the incidence of depression in women (Brown and Harris 1978). It has its basis in the lack of a warm confiding relationship that leads to feelings of vulnerability and lack of self-esteem or self-worth which makes support ineffective if not impossible. If unrelieved, these feelings lead to a degree of apathy and fear of further failure which renders women helpless and unable to change their situation.

Table 6.8 *EWB scores classified by life-crisis events* (Mann–Whitney *U* test corrected for ties)

Life-crisis	EWB	
	n	Mean rank score
Death of close family member		
Yes	61	123.6
No	211	132.4
	$z = 1.6177; P = 0.1057$	
Marriage changes		
Yes	37	123.6
No	233	137.4
	$z = -0.9988; P = 0.3179$	
Illness in close family		
Yes	66	128.9
No	205	138.3
	$z = -0.8464; P = 0.3973$	
Moved house		
Yes	112	125.4
No	160	144.3
	$z = -1.9461; P = 0.0516$	
Changes in husband's work		
Yes	90	120.9
No	173	137.9
	$z = -1.7009; P = 0.0890$	
Marital tension/giving up work		
Yes	90	115.1
No	181	146.4
	$z = -3.0953; P = 0.0020$	

Adjusting to giving up work

The other main area of conflict was reported by women who said they were finding difficulty in adjusting to being at home all day after giving up an interesting job and working environment. Several mothers commented about their feelings on this matter when they completed the post-natal questionnaire six weeks after the post-delivery interview. One commented:

> In spite of having a devoted and helpful husband I find loving our baby difficult still, and feel trapped when my husband goes out to work. I never realised how much freedom I'd lose having a baby.

Another mother, who had just left her post as a social worker, said:

> Being a mother is satisfying and totally exhausting and downgraded and not appreciated by our society!

Oakley (1980) argues that the primary loss in becoming a mother is loss of identity. Giving up an interesting and rewarding job is a loss of the mother's identity as a capable and valued member of the working population. Her competence in her chosen career is replaced at least initially by her 'apprenticeship' at the new job of motherhood. This loss of identity is made worse by a society which does not value the contribution made by all parents in their nurture of its future citizens. Leaving work also entails leaving the peer support of colleagues at a time when the opportunity to make new friends is restricted by the needs of a new baby.

Moving house

Women who moved house also suffered loss of identity and loss of peer support. The house is the woman's particular territory, the place where her personality and values have most expression and the place where she has primary control over the lifestyle of her family. The term 'housewife' is indicative of the way society identifies the role of women with the house in which they live in a way which would be unthinkable if applied to men. Moving house disrupts lifestyle and considerable effort and organisation is required before new patterns of living can be established. It also separates the mother from the support of family and friends in the area left behind, and this loss of support increases the likelihood that the mother's own needs will be submerged beneath those of her baby and the rest of her family to a considerable degree.

The life-events described above all increased the amount of stress with which the affected mothers were coping, by reducing the amount and quality of family or peer support which was available to them, and thus making them increasingly vulnerable to emotional distress.

The research design was based upon two hypotheses (see Chapter 4). The first hypothesis stated that:

> The emotional response of women to the changes which follow the birth of a child will be affected by their personality and by the quality of the support they receive from family and social support systems.

The analysis of the results discussed in this chapter upholds this hypothesis and illustrates the way in which factors in the mother and in her personal family situation affected her adjustment to motherhood.

The second hypothesis stated that:

> The way in which care is provided by midwives during the post-natal period will influence the emotional response of women to the changes which follow the birth of a child.

The study also identified factors which upheld the second hypothesis and which were related to the mother's feelings about her baby, her competence as a mother, and to the way in which care was given by midwives working in hospital.

Post-natal care factors which contributed to emotional well-being

The analysis of the results revealed two other factors which contributed to the vulnerability of mothers to depression. These were both identified from the mothers' assessments of the post-natal care received in hospital, and were maternal self-image in feeding and the amount of rest received during the stay in hospital.

A mother's score for these factors was significantly related to her EWB score but not to her personality trait nor to the degree of satisfaction she had with motherhood. Details are given in Table 6.9.

Table 6.9 EPI(N) scores, satisfaction with motherhood and EWB scores compared with scores for self-image in feeding and rest in hospital (Mann–Whitney U test corrected for ties)

	EPI(N)		Satisfaction with motherhood		EWB	
	n	Mean rank score	n	Mean rank score	n	Mean rank score
Self-image in feeding						
Low scores	62	132.1	61	132.1	63	93.0
Moderate/high scores	206	130.4	215	136.5	213	147.0
	$z = 1.5981; P = 0.1100$		$z = 1.3701; P = 0.1707$		$z = -3.7501; P = 0.0002$	
Rest in hospital						
Low scores	114	136.5	121	129.4	118	125.7
Moderate/high scores	154	133.0	156	143.5	161	150.5
	$z = 0.3619; P = 0.7174$		$z = -1.5572; P = 0.1192$		$z = -2.5297; P = 0.0114$	

Self-image in feeding

The self-image in feeding factor was quite separate from the feeding support factor, which reflected the mother's perception of the quality of support she received from midwives and other members of the nursing staff when feeding her baby. Instead it reflected her feelings and judgement of her own competence in feeding her baby compared with that of other mothers in the same ward (see pp. 42 and 43).

Depressed people are very self-critical and it might be considered that this was the reason for the strong relationship between low self-image in feeding scores and low EWB scores. There was, however, considerable evidence that this was not so, but that the self-image score reflected the mother's feelings during the early post-natal period rather than her feelings at the time when she completed the questionnaire.

The self-image in feeding scores were related to the mothers' level of experience of feeding a baby and to real difficulties which she encountered in feeding her baby and which were observed by the hospital midwives. The scores of primigravidae early in the post-natal period were accordingly significantly lower than those of the multiparous women, reflecting their lack of experience and competence in feeding a baby. Six weeks later, though, the EWB scores of primigravidae were not significantly different from those of the multiparae – in fact they were slightly higher.

The hospital midwives' reports confirmed the reality of the mother's feelings as revealed in her self-image in feeding score. During the interview held with a hospital midwife on the day each mother was discharged from hospital, the midwives had identified 54 mothers who had been 'unduly' distressed about feeding their babies and who had needed more than the 'normal' amount of help. Six weeks later these mothers scored significantly lower scores on the self-image in feeding factor than the rest of the sample.

Of these 54 mothers, 30 were breast feeding and 24 were bottle feeding their infants. The distressed mothers did not have higher EPI(N) scores than the rest of the sample, nor was the incidence of distress in feeding directly related to their EWB scores. Indeed the mean rank EWB scores of the 54 mothers seen to be distressed about feeding in hospital (mean rank = 135.1) was very similar to that of the remaining 211 mothers (mean rank = 138.1). Details can be seen in Table 6.10. (Information was missing from 10 mothers.)

Once again the picture emerges of two groups of mothers within the total group of those who had shown distress about feeding their babies in the early post-natal period. For many of them, initial anxiety was replaced by growing confidence and skill as they and their babies learnt together how to manage feeding. For others, the distress was a manifestation of continuing problems of low self-esteem, and continuing conflict.

A mother's self-image in feeding was also related to her perception of her baby's progress measured on the Broussard-type scale six weeks after delivery. Mothers were asked to assess whether their baby was better or worse than the 'average' baby in such matters as the number of crying spells, difficulties in feeding, sleeping difficulties and settling down to an expected pattern of behaviour. The concept of 'average' was that of the mother. Table 6.11 shows that 36 mothers thought their babies were doing worse than average on all four counts, 127 thought

Table 6.10 *EPI(N) scores and scores for self-image in feeding, rest in hospital, emotional well-being and satisfaction with motherhood classified by midwives' observations of maternal distress during feeding in the post-natal ward* (Mann–Whitney U test corrected for ties)

	Midwives' observations in post-natal ward	
Factors	Mothers distressed (mean rank scores; $n = 54$)	Mothers not distressed (mean rank scores; $n = 220$)
EPI(N)	127.8	133.0
	$z = -0.4438; P = 0.6572$	
Self-image in feeding	99.5	146.8
	$z = -3.9870; P = 0.0001$	
Rest in hospital	115.9	142.8
	$z = -2.2505; P = 0.0244$	
Emotional well-being	135.1	138.1
	$z = -0.2483; P = 0.8039$	
Satisfaction with motherhood	138.1	137.4
	$z = 0.0590; P = 0.9530$	

their baby was doing as well as the average baby and 112 said that their babies were doing better than the average baby. (Four mothers did not complete the score.) There were statistically significant differences in the self-image in feeding scores of the mothers in the three different groups, those who said their babies were doing worse than the average baby scoring the lowest self-image in feeding scores, and those who said their babies were doing better than average scoring much higher self-image in feeding scores (K–W test; $P = 0.0064$). The mother's self-image was affected by and affected her perception of her baby.

Implications of a low self-image in feeding score
The original study by Broussard and Hartner (1971) indicated that mothers with poor self-image regarded their babies as 'difficult' more often than did other mothers. Other studies have noted that low self-esteem in the mother is associated with problems in maternal–child relationships leading to child abuse (Lynch *et al*. 1976; Rosen and Stein 1980).

The study by Lynch *et al*. is particularly interesting because they found the same recognition of potential problems by mid-

Table 6.11 *EPI(N) scores and scores for self-image in feeding, emotional well-being and satisfaction with motherhood compared with the mother's perception of her six-week-old baby (Broussard-type score)* (Kruskall–Wallis one-way analysis of variance)

Factors	Mother said baby's progress was:		
	Worse than average (mean rank score; $n = 36$)	Average (mean rank score; $n = 127$)	Better than average (mean rank score; $n = 112$)
EPI(N)	141.7	132.2	128.6
		$\chi^2 = 0.7913; P = 0.6753$	
Self-image in feeding	117.3	127.6	155.1
		$\chi^2 = 10.0878; P = 0.0064$	
Emotional well-being	90.7	140.7	148.9
		$\chi^2 = 15.1281; P = 0.0005$	
Satisfaction with motherhood	103.3	135.8	150.4
		$\chi^2 = 9.9152; P = 0.0070$	

wives. The histories of women whose children had been referred
to the register of children at risk of non-accidental injury were
compared with those of controls whose babies had been born
in the same hospital and at the same time. It was found that
20 mothers whose children were on the At-Risk Register because
of neglect or abuse suffered from a number of interlocking marital and family problems over which they had little or no control
and that 72% of these mothers had been identified by the hospital midwives who cared for them as having problems in caring
adequately for and mothering their newborn babies. Lynch
noted that although these early difficulties in mothering had
been seen by the midwives, their potential as an early warning
of future problems had not been recognised. The recognition
by midwives in this study of problems associated with low
maternal self-image in feeding and poor perception of the baby's
progress six weeks after leaving the hospital confirm Lynch's
contention that the midwives' observations could be used to
identify serious potential problems in maternal–child relationships.

This picture of poor self-image which arose from and contributed to difficulties in important personal relationships is
reminiscent of Seligman's concept of 'learned helplessness'
(Seligman 1975), in which the victim copes by accepting a painful
situation as hopeless and ceases to make any effort to overcome
or avoid it. Seligman's studies showed that in the absence of
any other help, repeated failures in coping lead to apathy and
inaction. But he also had some success in reversing this pattern
by encouraging his subjects and enabling them to achieve small
successes until they began to believe that they could cope with
certain situations.

This possibility of effecting change in situations of apathy
and failure is most important when we consider the role and
practice of professional care-givers, whose purpose is to support
and enable those experiencing major change and stress to
triumph over it. Positive reinforcement and protection from
avoidable stress encourages coping behaviour, but negative reinforcement and exposure to unnecessary stress reduces confidence and frustrates the coping mechanism.

The present study revealed areas of negative reinforcement
and increased stress when a mother's score for self-image in

feeding was compared with her reactions to conflicting advice and insufficient rest in the hospital.

Conflicting advice
Conflicting advice was one of the major sources of dissatisfaction with post-natal care, especially among primigravidae (Ball 1984), and acted as a contributory factor in emotional distress. One hundred and nine mothers (39% of the total sample) complained about conflicting advice, and they scored significantly lower self-image in feeding scores than those who did not complain of it (M–W test; $P = 0.0024$).

For many of the mothers conflicting advice caused considerable distress:

> I was very annoyed that in hospital I didn't get enough help with the feeding. Before the birth everyone encourages breast feeding, but it seemed that for most of the staff it was too much trouble . . . much easier to give a bottle. By the time I left hospital I was totally confused and if it wasn't for the help and encouragement of the midwife at home I don't think I would have carried on.

Others found their own way of coping with it:

> I didn't seem to be able to do anything right, and then one midwife told me to feed the baby whenever he needed it, and another one told me off and said he shouldn't be fed more often than every three hours or else I would get sore nipples. In the end I didn't know what to do, and my mother said take no notice of them. In the end the nasty one went on her weekend off and I could manage all right and the feeding went well after that!

Although the majority of complaints about conflicting advice concerned the feeding of infants, they were not confined to it:

> All the mothers I spoke to also found the different and sometimes conflicting advice from the midwives confusing and upsetting. I heard two sisters tell one girl in my ward exactly opposite ways of folding cot sheets. This almost reduced her to tears as she was feeling depressed at the time. I felt it was unnecessary to make such an issue of so trivial a matter.

Many of the mothers were annoyed by conflicting advice but able to cope with the frustration it caused them. For others, however, it formed one more straw upon the camel's back contributing to the spiral of lowered self-esteem and emotional distress.

Lack of sleep in hospital

Another form of stress which affected the mother's self-image in feeding and her emotional well-being was lack of sleep in hospital.

One hundred and fourteen mothers recorded low scores for the rest in hospital factor, and these mothers also had significantly lower self-image in feeding (M–W test; $P = 0.0136$) and EWB scores (M–W test; $P = 0.0114$) than 161 mothers who recorded moderate or high scores for the rest in hospital factor. (No scores were available for 4 mothers.)

This factor was made up of three statements on the questionnaire about post-natal care in hospital. It was found that mothers in hospital 2 scored much higher levels of satisfaction with the rest factor than mothers in the other two hospitals. When the scores for the three statements which made up the factor were analysed by hospital it was found that there were no significant differences between hospitals for the statements 'It was easy to get enough rest in the day-time' (K–W test; $P = 0.1622$) and 'It was easy to relax and feel at home in the ward' (K–W test; $P = 0.2337$). But there were marked differences in the scores of the mothers in the three hospitals for the statement 'I needed more rest at night' (K–W test; $P = 0.0001$). It was therefore concluded that the main parameter operating within this factor was that related to the amount of rest at night.

A number of studies have shown that subjects deprived of the deeper stages of sleep rapidly become depressed and lethargic and lose their efficiency in carrying out their normal activities. They find it difficult to take in information, and have particular difficulty with learning and performing manual tasks. Studies of the effects of sleep deprivation show that sleep is an integral and vital part of the 24-hour biological cycle (Weinmann 1981).

It is therefore not surprising to find that the 54 mothers whom the midwives described as being unduly distressed about feeding their babies in the post-natal ward, recorded significantly lower scores for the rest factor six weeks later (M–W test; $P = 0.0244$) (see Table 6.10 above).

Altogether 116 mothers (41.6% of the total sample) had low scores on this factor, and those who were distressed about feeding accounted for almost half of them.

Important differences were found in the incidence of distress in feeding in the three hospitals, which provides further evidence of the relationship between lack of sleep and feeding difficulties. The mothers in hospital 2 scored significantly higher levels of satisfaction with the rest in hospital factor (K–W test; $P = 0.0030$) and the incidence of distress in feeding was significantly lower in this hospital than in the other two (chi-square $= 12.972767$; 4 d.f.; $P = 0.0116$). The self-image in feeding scores of mothers in hospital 2 were also significantly higher than those of mothers in the other hospitals (K–W test; $P = 0.0223$). There were no differences in the parity of the mothers in the three hospitals which might have accounted for these differences in the incidence of distress in feeding, nor were there any significant differences in anxiety rating (EPI(N) scores) which might have contributed towards sleep disturbance. Details can be seen in Table 6.12.

Table 6.12 *A comparison of the mothers' EPI(N) scores and scores for rest in hospital, self-image in feeding, emotional well-being and satisfaction with motherhood in the three hospitals* (Kruskall–Wallis one-way analysis of variance)

Factors	Hospital 1 (mean rank scores; $n = 112$)	Hospital 2 (mean rank scores; $n = 103$)	Hospital 3 (mean rank scores; $n = 63$)
EPI(N)	132.4	135.6	136.4
		$\chi^2 = 0.1412$; $P = 0.9318$	
Rest in hospital	132.6	160.3	119.7
		$\chi^2 = 11.6465$; $P = 0.0030$	
Self-image in feeding	128.8	157.0	131.9
		$\chi^2 = 7.6025$; $P = 0.0223$	
Emotional well-being	145.6	142.4	126.0
		$\chi^2 = 2.5252$; $P = 0.2829$	
Satisfaction with motherhood	141.0	143.8	131.9
		$\chi^2 = 0.9089$; $P = 0.6348$	

The differences in the mothers' scores for the rest in hospital factor and the effect which lack of sleep had upon their self-image in feeding and distress in feeding their babies were due to the different policies about the rooming-in of mothers and babies which operated in the three maternity hospitals. Rooming-in is the term given to the practice of keeping mothers and babies together as much as possible, and it has arisen as a result of studies of maternal–child relationships. (Klaus *et al.* 1972; Kennell *et al.* 1974; Leiderman and Seashore 1975). Many hospitals have adopted a policy of 24-hour rooming-in, believing that any separation of mother and baby must be harmful.

The evidence of lack of sleep and its effects arising from this study indicates that while the theoretical concepts behind rooming-in may be soundly based, the practice of it left much to be desired. Although the results of the studies listed above are frequently cited as a basis for 24-hour rooming-in, an examination of the major publication by Klaus and Kennell (*Parent–Infant Bonding*, 1982) reveals a recommendation that the baby should be kept at the mother's bedside for long periods in the day-time.

Hospital 2 had such a policy operating. For the first two days after delivery the babies were kept by their mothers' bedsides during the day from the time of the first feed in the morning until approximately 10 p.m. when they were taken into the ward nursery unless the mother particularly wanted her baby to remain with her during the night. They were then brought to their mothers for feeding during the night. On the third day the mothers were invited to have their babies with them throughout the 24 hours if they wished. The majority of them (69%) went home during the third day, and many of those who remained, elected to continue the previous pattern of the baby sleeping in the nursery and being brought to them for feeding. As a result there were very few babies in the ward during the night.

In hospitals 1 and 3 the policy was that the babies were cared for in the ward nursery for the first night after delivery and then remained at the mother's bedside 24 hours a day. There were numerous complaints about the policies of rooming-in by the mothers in the hospitals concerned. It was not unusual for mothers to have their babies left with them throughout the first night after delivery.

One mother recalled that after several hours in labour her baby had been born in the early hours of the morning. That same night the baby was left by her bedside:

> All that night she cried continuously; no-one came to see if I needed any help. I felt so distraught . . . and was so tired I was afraid of dropping the baby. Finally at 2 a.m. I had to get up and ask if someone would look after my baby so that I could get some sleep.

Another mother was put in a four-bedded ward with three ante-natal mothers who had been admitted for rest:

> I was in a ward with three expectant mothers and I was the only one with a baby, so at his every whimper I was awake so that he wouldn't wake the others. After three days and nights with very little sleep I asked if the baby could go into the nursery just so I could get some sleep, but I was told the nursery was full with newborn babies.

It should be remembered that these comments were written by mothers six weeks after they had gone home from hospital, and they indicate the strong feelings mothers had about this matter. They also illustrate poor management of care by midwives on night duty, some of whom said that hospital policy did not allow them to take the babies out of the wards at night.

Lack of sleep is a frequent complaint of hospital patients, who find it difficult to settle in a strange environment and are disturbed by noise and lights. Disturbance is even more likely in any ward with newborn babies crying during the night. In a study of feeding and crying patterns of the newborn, Bernal (1972) noted that there was a peak of crying between midnight and 6 a.m. Many surveys of maternal satisfaction with post-natal care reveal a high degree of complaint about the lack of sleep caused by rooming-in policies. Clayton (1979) found that 47% of the mothers in a modern maternity hospital complained of too little sleep because of rooming-in, and a study of post-natal care by Filshie *et al.* (1981) found that 81% of mothers nursed in four-bedded wards complained of lack of sleep. The 'That's Life' survey (Boyd and Sellers 1982) collected the opinions of 6000 self-elected mothers and found that many women did not want the baby to be with them throughout the night but particularly liked the arrangement where babies stayed in the nursery at night and mothers were woken to feed them. A comparative study by Cox (1974) found that 40% of the mothers whose babies stayed with them during the night from 48 hours after the birth complained of too little sleep. In a controlled study in the USA Draramraj *et al.* (1981) found that although certain groups of mothers certainly desired and appreciated 24-hour rooming-in, this opinion was by no means universal and that the factors which influenced the mothers' choice of whether to room-in or not varied among different groups of mothers. Cox and Draramraj both concluded that maternal choice should be the deciding factor in the matter.

It is unfortunate that in spite of all the evidence that mothers find 24-hour rooming-in troublesome, many maternity hospitals still practise the policy in a routine and indiscriminate manner.

The effects which conflicting advice and lack of sleep in hospital had upon the mothers' self-image and emotional well-being, uphold the second hypothesis that the way in which post-natal care is provided by midwives will affect the mother's emotional response to the changes which follow the birth of a child.

Satisfaction with motherhood

The results discussed thus far in this chapter show how a mother's post-natal emotional well-being is affected by her personality and by a number of other stresses which make her vulnerable to emotional distress. There was, however, a third parameter in this interactive process and this had the effect of enriching the emotional response of the mother in such a way that she was enabled to overcome many of the difficulties which beset her. This parameter was the mother's satisfaction with motherhood, which was an outgoing emotion directed towards the baby rather than a reflection of the mother's internal emotional state.

Satisfaction with motherhood was measured by the mother's score on the satisfaction with motherhood factor – the second to emerge from the factor analysis of the emotional well-being questionnaire. This factor contained five statements which expressed the mother's feelings towards her baby. The possible range of scores was from 5 to 25, and the actual range of scores recorded by the mothers was from 14 to 25, with a mean average of 20.656 and a standard deviation of 2.410. This range of scores indicates the very positive pattern of scoring for this factor.

Only 3 mothers (1.1%) recorded a score of 14 (equal to a mean average of less than 2.8 per statement), and these women were considered to have low satisfaction with motherhood. Seventy-seven mothers (27.6%) scored between 15 and 19 (equal to a mean average of 3–3.95 per statement) and this group was classed as having moderate satisfaction with motherhood. The remaining 199 mothers (71.3%) recorded scores of 20 or more (equal to a mean average of at least 4 per statement) and were considered to have very high satisfaction with motherhood.

A positive relationship was found between the mother's satisfaction with motherhood and her emotional well-being scores, the details of which can be seen in Table 6.13.

Although the small number in the low satisfaction group is likely to have distorted the results of the one-way analysis of variance, analysis by Spearman rank correlation also revealed a significant relationship between the scores for satisfaction with motherhood and emotional well-being of the 216 mothers in

Table 6.13 *EWB scores compared with scores for satisfaction with motherhood*

(a) Kruskall–Wallis one-way analysis of variance		
Satisfaction with motherhood	**EWB**	
	n	Mean rank score
Low scores	3	33.8
Moderate scores	77	124.7
High scores	199	147.5
	$\chi^2 = 9.7071; P = 0.0078$	

(b) Spearman rank correlation			
Satisfaction with motherhood of mothers in:		**EWB**	
	n	Spearman rank correlation	Significance
Hospital 1	112	0.3532	$P = 0.001$
Hospital 2	104	0.5557	$P = 0.001$
Hospital 3	63	−0.1650	Not significant

hospitals 1 and 2. This relationship was further confirmed by multiple regression analysis of the total sample, which will be discussed later.

As the overwhelming majority of mothers expressed high satisfaction with motherhood it would seem that the mother's joy and delight in her baby made a positive contribution to her emotional well-being, boosting her morale and enriching the adjustment process.

Further analysis revealed that the mother's feelings immediately after the birth of her baby (which were recorded within 24 – 36 hours of the birth) were closely linked to her degree of satisfaction with motherhood six weeks later (see Table 6.18 below), and that these feelings did not appear to have been affected by trait anxiety or eroded by other factors and events which have been shown to have an adverse effect upon post-natal emotional well-being.

The degree of trait anxiety in the maternal personality – which had such a marked effect on her emotional well-being, self-confidence, and perception of hospital care and family support – did not have a similar effect on satisfaction with motherhood (see Table 6.14).

Mothers who had a low score for self-image in feeding, and those who were seen to be distressed about feeding their infants whilst in hospital, did not score any less satisfaction with motherhood than other mothers (see Tables 6.9 and 6.10 above).

Although lack of rest in hospital was related to the patterns of rooming-in of babies and mothers, and had an effect on emotional well-being, it did not have a similar effect on satisfaction with motherhood (see Table 6.9 above) and there were no

Table 6.14 *EPI(N) scores compared with scores for satisfaction with motherhood*

Satisfaction with motherhood	EPI(N)	
	n	Mean rank scores
Low scores	3	143.0
Moderate scores	75	128.1
High scores	190	136.9
	$\chi^2 = 0.7350; P = 0.6925$	

significant differences in the satisfaction with motherhood of the mothers in the three different hospitals (see Table 6.12 above). This indicates that the practice of putting babies in the nursery at night did not have a detrimental effect upon the developing relationship between the mother and her baby.

Mothers who bottle fed their infants did not record any less satisfaction with motherhood than breast feeding mothers, and there was no evidence that the mother's age or parity had any significant effect upon her satisfaction with motherhood (see Table 6.15).

All these results lead one to conclude that satisfaction with motherhood is a distinct and stable matrix of feelings and motivation.

Relationship with the mother's feelings immediately after the birth

These feelings were also expressed in the mother's reactions immediately after the birth of the baby, and a highly significant relationship was found between the mother's reported feelings at that time and her satisfaction with motherhood six weeks later (see Table 6.16). The details of the interview in which the mother recorded these feelings are given in Chapter 4.

Table 6.15 *Scores for satisfaction with motherhood classified by age, parity, and choice of feeding method*

	Satisfaction with motherhood	
Variable	n	Mean rank scores
Age of mother		
17–20 years	31	146.4
21–29 years	164	135.3
30–39 years	84	146.8
K–W test:	$\chi^2 = -1.3637; P = 0.5057$	
Parity		
Primigravidae	98	144.2
Multiparae	179	136.1
M–W test:	$z = 0.8097; P = 0.4181$	
Choice of feeding method		
Breast	161	141.0
Bottle	112	131.2
M–W test:	$z = 1.0238; P = 0.3059$	

It can be seen in Table 6.16 that the 6 mothers who said that they were 'disappointed' and the 19 who said that they felt 'too tired to care' scored the lowest levels of satisfaction with motherhood, and that the highest level of satisfaction was recorded by the 71 mothers who said that they had felt 'gloriously happy' immediately after the birth of the baby.

There is some evidence that mothers who were highly motivated towards motherhood before delivery scored more positive feelings immediately after the baby's birth, and that mothers who fed their newborn infants during the first hour after delivery also recalled more positive feelings. There was no evidence that the type of labour or delivery affected the mothers' feelings immediately afterwards (see Table 6.17).

During the ante-natal interview 67 women had expressed their eager anticipation of becoming mothers, some of them for the second or third time, and these women later expressed much more positive feelings after the birth.

It appears that the mother's attention immediately after the birth was centred upon her newborn infant and her feelings towards him or her, rather than the events of labour and delivery which had resulted in the birth. It is therefore not surprising to find that the giving and receiving of a feed enhanced the mother's pleasure in her achievement.

Table 6.16 *Scores for satisfaction with motherhood compared with mothers' reported feelings after delivery* (Kruskall–Wallis one-way analysis of variance)

| Feelings after delivery[a] | Satisfaction with motherhood[b] | |
	n	Mean rank score
Disappointed	6	76.3
Too tired to care	19	105.3
Relieved	82	125.9
Tired and happy	83	110.7
Gloriously happy	71	172.2
	$\chi^2 = 33.4957; P = 0.0001$	

[a] Recorded within 24–36 hours of the birth. Fourteen mothers gave no definite answer and are not included.
[b] Recorded 6–8 weeks after the birth.

*Effect on satisfaction with motherhood of feeding the baby
in the first hour after delivery*

Mothers who fed their babies during the first hour after delivery recalled more positive feelings at that time and the highest levels of satisfaction with motherhood six weeks later (see Table 6.18).

A number of studies have focused upon the contact between the mother and her baby during the first hour after delivery, and have demonstrated the beneficial effect which a period of mutual physical contact has upon the developing maternal–child relationship. When a baby is held in the *en face* position he or she is able to gaze into the mother's eyes, and this creates a deep bond between them. It has also been observed that when mothers are left alone with their newborn infants they follow a particular pattern of exploring the baby's body (Klaus *et al.* 1972, 1975; Leiderman and Seashore 1975; Klaus and Kennell 1970, 1976, 1982). The giving of a feed allows a mother to have a period of uninterrupted time with her baby during the first hour after the birth, and appears to assume a pivotal position between her experience of labour and delivery and her outward and infant-directed feelings of joy and satisfaction with motherhood.

Table 6.17 *Scores for birth feelings classified by type of labour and delivery*

		Birth feelings	
Variable	*n*	Mean rank score	
Type of labour			
Spontaneous	121	131.6	
Induced	97	148.4	
Active Management	58	136.3	
		$\chi^2 = 2.6064; P = 0.2717$	
Type of delivery			
Normal	194	137.7	
Forceps	49	133.1	
Breech	4	161.8	
Caesarian section	29	149.8	
		$\chi^2 = 1.2556; P = 0.7397$	

It might be supposed that mothers who had a difficult delivery would be less likely to feed their babies, but this was not so. Forty per cent of the women who had a forceps delivery fed their babies during the first hour compared with 45% of those who had a normal delivery. Two of the four women who had a breech delivery fed their babies, and three of the mothers who had a caesarian section under epidural analgesia fed their babies whilst still in the operating theatre. It would appear that whether or not a mother fed her baby during the first hour after birth depended upon her choice of breast or bottle feeding, and upon the management of care in the delivery suite.

One hundred and thirteen mothers (40.5% of the total sample) fed their babies during the first hour, and of these 107 breast fed their babies and 6 bottle fed. All the hospitals had policies which said that mothers should be encouraged to put the baby to the breast as soon as possible after birth, the main purpose behind the policy being the need for the stimulation of lactation in mothers who intended to breast feed. The enrichment of the maternal–child relationship which suckling a baby also brings

Table 6.18 *Scores for birth feelings and satisfaction with motherhood classified by time of first feed to infant* (Mann–Whitney U test corrected for ties)

(a)　　Birth feelings		
	Birth feelings (24 hours after birth)	
Time of first feed	n	Mean rank score
Within 1 hour of birth	112	153.3
More than 1 hour after birth	164	129.8
	$z = 2.2769$; $P = 0.0228$	

(b)　　Satisfaction with motherhood		
	Satisfaction with motherhood (6 weeks after birth)	
Time of first feed	n	Mean rank score
Within 1 hour of birth	113	151.6
More than 1 hour after birth	165	131.2
	$z = 2.0921$; $P = 0.0364$	

seemed to be overlooked. However, even though such policies were in existence, it was found that 76 of the 183 mothers who had elected to breast feed did not put their babies to the breast at this time.

As the study did not include observing the birth of the baby, it is not possible to ascertain all the events which led to a mother feeding or not feeding her baby. However, there is some evidence to suggest that the more articulate mothers were given a greater opportunity to feed their babies. Although allowance must be made for the social class differences in the choice of breast or bottle feeding, it is notable that 60% of those who fed their babies came from social classes 1, 2 and 3n/m, and only 40% from social classes 3m, 4 and 5. Mothers aged between 21 and 29 years formed 62% of those who fed their babies. Ten mothers aged under 20 elected to breast feed but only three of them fed their babies during the first hour after the birth.

Attention must also be called to the needs of mothers who chose to bottle feed, as it is these women who were most deprived of the opportunity which the giving of a feed provided for the mother and her baby to be left alone together. It is in the giving and receiving of a feed that maternal–child relationships are enriched, and it is to be regretted that mothers who choose to bottle feed are rarely given an opportunity to do so shortly after the baby's birth. Indeed it may be some time before mother and baby enjoy a feed together in the post-natal ward. The same *en face* position that the baby automatically assumes when held to suckle at the breast can also be achieved when the baby is held in the mother's arms to bottle feed.

As the giving of a feed was associated with positive feelings immediately after delivery and increased satisfaction with motherhood six weeks later, it is likely that careful management of post-delivery care, which ensures that every mother and baby spend a period of time together, would enrich the experience of motherhood and, by its reinforcement of the mother's feelings towards her baby, could make a positive contribution to her emotional well-being.

Conclusions

The results of the present study show that maternal emotional well-being measured six weeks after the birth of the baby was

significantly affected by or associated with three interacting sets
of factors, which are illustrated in Figs. 6.1 and 6.2.

Fig. 6.1 illustrates maternal and family factors which formed
a pattern of vulnerability; most have been identified in previous
studies of distress and depression. These were the effects of
anxiety (Tod 1964; Pitt 1968; Wilson-Barnett 1979), loss of identity
(Dalton 1980; Oakley 1980), and the lack of a warm confiding
relationship with the husband or male partner (Stott 1973;
Brown and Harris 1978). These factors had a marked effect upon
the mother's emotional well-being but were not associated with
her satisfaction with motherhood or her perception of her 6-
week-old infant's progress.

Fig. 6.1 Antecedent factors related to emotional well-being and
satisfaction with motherhood six weeks after the birth.

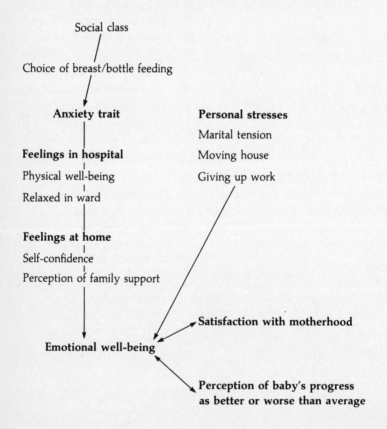

A different set of factors is seen in Fig. 6.2. These fall into two main groups, both of which were affected to some degree by post-natal care. The first group links the mother's recorded feelings immediately after the birth, her satisfaction with motherhood and her perception of the baby's progress, all of which were directly related to emotional well-being. The second group surrounds the mother's self-image in feeding in the early days after the birth of the baby, and this was related to her emotional well-being and to her perception of the baby's progress six weeks later, but not to her satisfaction with motherhood.

Low self-esteem is a symptom of depression (Seligman 1975), and it might have been assumed that this factor was entirely due to the mother's emotional state when she completed the questionnaire six weeks after the birth of the baby. But this

Fig. 6.2 Other factors related to emotional well-being and satisfaction with motherhood six weeks after the birth.

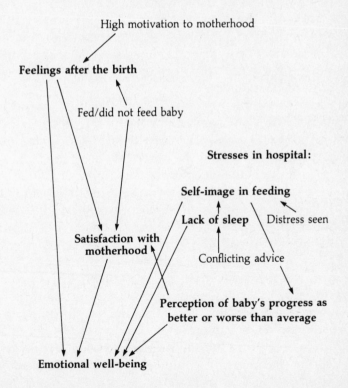

assumption cannot be sustained in the light of other evidence. Primigravidae recorded lower self-image in feeding scores six weeks after the birth, but they were not more emotionally distressed than multiparous women at that time, and the hospital midwives identified those mothers whose distress in feeding their babies later resulted in low scores for self-image in feeding. Self-image in feeding was adversely affected by the increased stress which arose from conflicting advice and from lack of sleep during the mother's stay in hospital.

In order to determine the degree to which these different factors combined together to affect post-natal emotional outcome, a further analysis was undertaken using multiple regression. This technique examines the degree to which differences in a group of significant variables affect the dependent variable (Stopher and Meyburg 1979).

A number of analyses were carried out, using both the stepwise and direct forms of regression. The full range of maternal scores for emotional well-being were tested against the mother's anxiety score on the Eysenck Personality Inventory (EPI(N) score), the birth feelings scores, all the post-natal care factor scores, the satisfaction with motherhood scores and the mother's perception of her baby's progress measured by her scores on the Broussard-type scale.

The highest multiple regression score (multiple $R = 0.70746$) was obtained when the combined effect of the group of factors shown in Table 6.19 was analysed. The factors are listed in the table in the order in which they are shown by the regression to have had a predictive effect upon emotional outcome.

The consistent relationship between personality and emotional well-being is seen in the presence of the EPI(N) scores and in four other factors which also related to the mother's degree of anxiety. The EPI(N) score which was recorded approximately four weeks before the baby was born is placed sixth in relation to the mother's emotional well-being when her baby was six weeks old. The degree of anxiety in a mother's personality also affected her ability to relax and feel at home in the post-natal ward (eighth in order), her perception of family support (fifth in order) and her self-confidence when she first came home (second in order). Its continuing effect is seen in the first factor listed in the predictive order, which was the mother's

perception of the quality of the support she was recei
her family at the time when she filled in the questic

The less anxious women were coping quite well and ю.
the help they were receiving was sufficient for their needs, but
the scores of the distressed women constituted a cry for help.
They were not yet able to cope alone and felt that they needed
more help than they were receiving. Although the results show
that anxiety played a large part in their perceptions, these scores
also call into question the assumption that a woman 'ought' to
be able to cope with all the demands of the household by the
time her baby is six weeks old.

The remaining factors listed were not related to the mother's
personality but arose from her feelings towards her baby and

Table 6.19 *Multiple regression analysis of major factors related to post-natal emotional well-being*

Dependent variable: emotional well-being

Mean response	78.34601	Standard deviation	11.45078
Multiple R	0.70746	Analysis of variance	DF
R square	0.50049	Regression	8
Adjusted R square	0.48476	Residual	254
S.D.	8.21938	Coefficient of variability	10.5%

$F = 31.81283$; Level of significance = 0.0001

Variable	B coefficient	S.E. of B	F/Significance
Family support (six weeks post-partum)	1.2460546	0.24199185	25.513844/ 0.0001
Self-confidence (1–2 weeks post-partum)	1.1396136	0.31803888	12.839698/ 0.0001
Broussard-type score (6 weeks post-partum)	1.1197801	0.58280626	3.6916206/ 0.056
Self-image in feeding	0.67895392	0.25635193	7.0146730/ 0.009
Family support (1–2 weeks post-partum)	0.67188137	0.24073798	7.7892556/ 0.006
EPI(N) score (36 weeks pregnant)	−0.59274737	0.12135500	23.857445 0.0001
Satisfaction with motherhood (6 weeks post-partum)	0.52256611	0.22479123	5.4041040 0.021
Ward atmosphere (1 week post-partum)	0.31435893	0.16352195	3.6957235 0.056

about her own competence in mothering, and were affected to a certain degree by the care she received from midwives.

The Broussard-type score was listed third in the predictive order and its relationship to both emotional well-being and satisfaction with motherhood suggest that it was a powerful indicator of the mother's feelings and perceptions six weeks after the birth of the baby.

The mother's score on this scale was closely associated with her score for self-image in feeding, which is fourth in the predictive order and which was affected by stress in the post-natal ward.

Satisfaction with motherhood, which acted as a boost to the mother's emotional state, was listed seventh, indicating the significance of its contribution to the adjustment process.

The results of the study and the interaction of significant factors shown in the results of the multiple regression analysis upheld both hypotheses. The mother's personality and the quality of her family and social support certainly affected her response to the changes which resulted from the birth of her baby, and the way that midwives cared for the mother during the post-natal period also had a significant effect upon her well-being.

7

'Loading the dice': interaction of personal needs and support systems

The results of the study illustrate the way in which a woman's adjustment to motherhood is influenced by a number of factors which interact with each other in a complex and dynamic manner.

Although the outcome of the coping process is strongly influenced by personality and previous experience, coping behaviour is also modified by the attitudes and expectations of peers and of the society to which the stressed person belongs. The way in which a person reacts to stress and change, therefore, is the result of an interaction between that person's internal needs, the amount of stress which is being experienced, and the quality of the supportive environment (Lazarus 1966, 1969; Caplan 1969; Caplan and Killilea 1976; Derlega and Janda 1978).

The supportive environment which surrounds mothers is composed of the help they receive from family and friends, and the help provided by society in the form of maternity and social services. The effectiveness of that support will depend upon the quality of the relationships which exist within the family and between the mother and her peers, and upon the degree of skills, understanding and resources provided by professional and other care-givers who have a particular role to play in the maternity services. The influence which professional and other care-givers can have upon patterns of coping and adjustment is highlighted by Caplan (1969). He believes that although the coping response is mainly determined by the individual's personality, and by his or her physiological and social characteristics, the intervention of care-givers may 'load the dice' and lead to an outcome which is either better or worse than might have been expected.

These patterns of vulnerability, coping and support described by Lazarus and Caplan can be clearly seen in the results which have been described in the previous chapter, and the interaction between the various factors in this process is illustrated by the findings of the multiple regression analysis.

Interacting factors in adjustment to motherhood

The multiple regression analysis produced a list of eight factors whose combined effect had the most impact upon emotional outcome for the mothers in the study. These factors, which are shown in Table 6.19 (p.115), are listed below in order of their cumulative effect upon emotional outcome. Good scores on all these factors would result in a high degree of emotional well-being, while poor scores on all of them would result in considerable distress. But as these factors also interact with each other, if poor scores on certain factors were counterbalanced by good scores on others, it might be possible for the potential emotional outcome to be improved.

Factors associated with different levels of maternal emotional well-being six weeks after the birth of the baby were:

*1. Perception of family support six weeks after delivery
*2. Mother's self-confidence when she first returned home with the baby (first week after delivery)
3. Mother's rating of her baby's progress in relation to her concept of the 'average' baby (Broussard-type scale six weeks after delivery)
4. Mother's self-image in feeding her baby during her stay in hospital (first seven days after delivery)
*5. Perception of family support when the mother first returned home with the baby (first week after delivery)
*6. Anxiety trait score on the Eysenck Personality Inventory (approximately four weeks before delivery)
7. Satisfaction with motherhood six weeks after delivery
*8. Reaction to post-natal ward atmosphere (first seven days after delivery)

The scores on those factors marked with an asterisk were closely related to the mother's score on the anxiety trait scale of the Eysenck Personality Inventory.

The results of the analysis point the way in which post-natal care could be changed in order to improve the potential emo-

of society change. It should not be rigid, nor should it assume that the same amount of support is needed by all mothers irrespective of their circumstances.

The potential of this interactive framework is perhaps best illustrated by the story of Janet, who was one of the mothers who gave birth in hospital 3. Her story shows the way in which a number of factors which made Janet vulnerable to emotional distress were counteracted by the sympathy of her obstetrician, the help of her husband and a close friend, and by the care of a 'smashing' midwife.

When Janet returned her post-natal questionnaire, the back of each page was covered with her description of her mothering situation and how she felt about it.

Janet's story

Janet was a married woman of 28 years, pregnant for the second time. The pregnancy was not planned. Her first child was a boy of 8 years, who had been born by caesarian section. In the ante-natal interview Janet had expressed great fear about the possibility of another caesarian section. Her anxiety score on the Eysenck Personality Inventory was high; her extroversion/ introversion score was average.

Janet's husband had recently become unemployed; his previous job had been that of a truck driver. Janet had been working as a bakery operative until 6 weeks before her baby was born.

The family was experiencing considerable financial problems which had begun when Janet's husband lost his job, and had not been improved by a serious fire which had damaged their council flat four months previously. This had been due to faulty wiring, for which the council had taken responsibility. However, the council had told Janet and her husband that the re-decoration of the flat could not be undertaken for at least six months. As the new baby was due before that time, the couple had undertaken the work themselves, but the council then refused to meet the costs because they said that Janet and her husband should have waited for them to do it. This argument had not been resolved by the time the baby was actually born, and Janet and her husband had got into arrears with the rent.

tional outcome. Although those factors associated with anxiety trait may not be readily amenable to change, those related to the management of care obviously are.

Five of the factors were related to *trait anxiety,* which is a stable personality trait. Many psychologists believe, however, that major life experiences can influence personality (Erikson 1959, 1963; Mischel 1968). It is important, therefore, that a woman's experience of childbirth and motherhood is one which enriches her psychological strengths as much as possible, and the caregiver should not lose sight of the fact that a good experience can boost a woman's confidence in herself to a considerable degree.

Trait anxiety affected the mother's perception and reactions in hospital and her self-confidence when she returned home. The effects of high anxiety upon patient's reactions to hospital and to certain procedures has been explored by Wilson-Barnett (1979), whose work provides a useful review of methods which can help all care-givers, including midwives, to recognise and alleviate some of the effects of anxiety.

The remaining factors were related to the mother's feelings about her baby and to her confidence as a mother.

Satisfaction with motherhood acted as a boost to maternal emotional well-being; it was manifest in the mother's reported feelings immediately after the birth and was enhanced by feeding the baby at that time. The relationships between midwives and mothers, and their husbands if present, are very close at the time surrounding the birth. They have shared the experience of labour and delivery together and even when the midwife has not personally conducted the delivery, she is the one who cares for the mother and baby immediately afterwards. Midwives therefore have a great opportunity to enhance the relationship between the mother and her baby at this particular time, by encouraging the mother to handle her baby, to feed him and to delight in him. This is particularly important when the mother appears to be indifferent towards her baby, and it may be necessary for the midwife to spend a longer time with such a mother in order to encourage her to respond to her baby.

Self-image in feeding was the fourth most important factor in terms of its effect on emotional outcome, and is the factor most amenable to change. Midwives were able to identify mothers who were experiencing distress, and it is therefore possible for their perceptions to be harnessed for the mothers' benefit.

Conflicting advice arises from uncoordinated delivery of care, and is a problem which must be overcome. It could be reduced if all professional care-givers involved with new mothers – doctors, midwives and health visitors – were a little more gracious of their colleagues' advice and refrained from contradicting it unless there was very good reason. This could be achieved by a team approach to the care of mothers in a post-natal ward, and by ensuring clear communications between the community midwife and health visitor.

Increased rest in hospital could be achieved by reducing the amount of disturbance caused by crying babies at night, and by enabling mothers to rest during the day-time.

The mother's self-image in feeding and her satisfaction with motherhood were both linked to feeding her baby, and both were related to the mother's score on the Broussard-type scale which recorded her perception of the baby's progress six weeks after the birth. The Broussard-type scale proved to be a powerful indicator of the mother's feelings about herself and about her baby, and could be used to identify vulnerable women in order to give them special care before the spiral of distress, disappointment and a deteriorating maternal–child relationship gets out of control.

The support system deckchair

Post-natal care is one part of the whole interactive framework of support which a woman needs if she is to make a successful and happy adjustment to motherhood. This interactive framework is illustrated in Fig. 7.1, which might be termed the 'support system deckchair'. If a deckchair is not erected properly, it will collapse under the weight of its occupant; if it does not stand upon a firm base it will fall over with similar results; and if the parts do not fit together well the occupant may be held up, but will become uncomfortable and strained. The emotional well-being of mothers and babies hangs on the framework of their individual support system as does the seat from the frame of a deckchair.

The mother's personality and her previous experien largely fixed and impervious to change, so are represer the fixed and rigid strut of the chair. The first and para support is that provided by the mother's husband, fam friends, which is therefore represented by the main sup strut. The bottom strut of any deckchair is notched in allow its occupant varying degrees of support; represen maternity services by this strut illustrates the need for be flexible enough to provide support as required by two parts of the framework. Finally, the whole structu upon the attitudes and values of society and the resource it provides for the care of mothers and families. Any support system needs to be adaptable and capable of c as women's needs and expectations change, and as the a

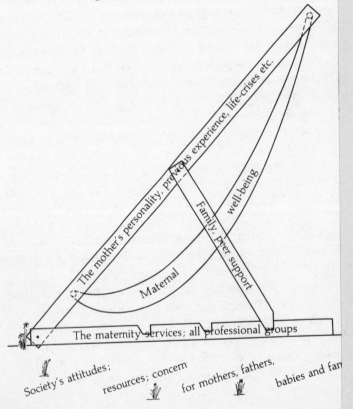

Fig. 7.1. The support system 'deck-chair'.

Janet was allowed to go into normal labour in the hope that she could deliver her baby vaginally, but this did not prove possible and after eight hours of labour she gave birth to another son, Daniel, by caesarian section under general anaesthetic. The baby's condition at birth was excellent. Janet chose to bottle feed her baby and did not give him a feed herself until he was over 24 hours old.

The post-natal ward staff noticed that Janet seemed to be distressed about feeding her baby and considered that this was due to discomfort after the caesarian section. They also noted that she was tearful, not sleeping well, and somewhat irritable during her stay in hospital.

Janet comments on her hospital care:

> It is difficult to answer about being fit and well, because I did feel well really, except that I had a terrible problem with wind. None of the nurses or doctors seemed to know how bad it was; they kept giving me some white stuff which did no good at all. It was only when I couldn't stand it any longer after two whole days without sleep because of the pain, that they took any notice, and they only took notice because I was crying. They gave me some suppositories and they didn't work very well either. In the end I got rid of it myself with experience, bending up and down. The relief was so great I skipped back to bed. Other than that I felt perfectly well. The only other thing that spoiled my stay in hospital was the food – it was awful. I got my husband and sister to bring me in sandwiches because I was starving. And the rules over staying up and watching televison. I think they aren't fair at all – they make you feel as though you are in prison or something, saying you've got to go to bed at a certain time. Hospital is boring enough so I think you should have something to look forward to even if it's only the late film.

Janet went home when the baby was seven days old. She writes about her experiences then:

> After I arrived home I did find it difficult to rest, but with the help of my husband and a very good friend

who lives around the corner I seemed to manage. My friend Pauline told me I looked very tired and so that I could sleep she took the baby for a whole day. It was the best sleep I had for a long time. Don't get me wrong, baby Daniel was very good, but I was conscious that he was there and that I must wake up every four hours for him. I'm still nervous now if he sleeps for a long time because I'm frightened of him dying from cot death and if anything happened to him now I don't know what I'd do. Some people have different ideas about letting babies sleep. The nurses say don't let him sleep longer than six hours, and older women I've talked to say let him sleep, he'll wake when he wants to, but I wake him up –I'm not taking any chances.

The midwives who came to see me were marvellous, especially the one who came all the time. She used to ask me all about the baby and myself, and seemed really concerned. I really looked forward to her coming for a chat and advice. She never seemed to be in a hurry, she was a smashing lady. She seemed more like a mother to me and always told me off if she found I'd been doing housework. I didn't need to do anything at all, I had more than enough help, but I don't like putting on people.

She discusses how she feels now that Daniel is six weeks old:
In answer to number 7 [on the emotional well-being questionnaire] I do get upset easily, I don't know why. My husband says I snap at him for the least little thing but he says he understands. I also get weepy but mostly when I'm on my own.

I talk to the baby all the time. He's gorgeous and now he's talking back to me and saying agoo, and he's nearly always smiling. I'd do anything for him when he smiles and tries to talk back to me, he makes me feel all excited.

When my first baby was born, I was 19 years old and my husband was 18. I was very poorly having him and sure that if I ever had to have another section I would kill myself. When I found I was having another one with Daniel I told my husband to take the baby and leave me because I didn't think I'd live through it, but everything was fine. On my first baby the nurse took all my jewellery off me and put it in a brown envelope. I had bad dreams all during the operation, and I dreamt that my husband came to the hospital and all they gave him was this brown envelope, yet on this second operation they just covered my jewellery with plaster and I had no bad dreams.

The reason I mentioned our ages is because I think that we were too young to have a baby then. My husband never helped me hardly at all, he just didn't seem interested in the baby, yet this time he feeds the baby and always wakes up when he's crying. And he's even changed him a few times – one thing I thought he'd never do. In fact I'm very proud of him. As we've gotten older I think we've become more settled and going out doesn't bother us like it did nine years ago.

Sometimes I do feel that the baby doesn't belong to me. It's hard to get used to having a baby really after waiting eight years since my other little boy.

After my first baby when I went for the coil the doctor asked me if I wanted more babies, and as I really wanted a girl I said yes. He said that if I had the coil I would probably never conceive again but he didn't say why. Therefore I didn't have the coil and I was poorly on the pill. All that was left was the sheath and that kept bursting and I was frightened because I was told you had a bad time if you got pregnant that way. I think that had a lot to do with feeling that my baby isn't mine is because I thought I would never have another, and with a caesarian one minute he's inside and the next he's out – you don't see him being born – so you don't feel he's yours at first. But both boys look so like their father that I know they're mine and I can see that they're mine.

I know that my baby knows that I love him by the way he looks at me and smiles – his eyes are full of love. If he wakes up crying in his pram and I call his name and go to him, he smiles and gets excited, because he knows I love him very much. I love kissing the back of his neck and feeling his bottom. I love when he is in the nude and I can feel his lovely warm body next to mine. His skin feels beautiful.

The lessons from Janet's story

It can be seen that there were a number of factors which 'loaded the dice' for Janet and made her a potential candidate for emotional distress.

The events of her previous pregnancy and caesarian section had left her with a great dread of repeating the experience. The pregnancy was unplanned, and Janet says that she was convinced she would die if she had another caesarian section. She recounts how young and immature she and her husband were at the time of the older boy's birth.

Janet had a high degree of anxiety trait in her personality and she and her husband had recently faced a number of stressful life-events. She did not feed Daniel until 24 hours after his birth, and she did not feel relaxed or at home in the hospital situation.

These loading factors were counteracted by the kind of support Janet received, and the growing maturity of Janet and her husband.

The obstetrician who cared for Janet was very sympathetic to her fears, and made every endeavour to enable Janet to have a vaginal delivery for her second baby. The trust which had grown between them enabled Janet to face the second operation and to find it an altogether different experience from the first. Her friend Pauline seemed to have had a great deal of common sense and stepped in with an offer of help at just the right moment.

It is obvious that Janet felt that her community midwife cared about her as an individual, was unhurried, friendly and approachable: 'She seemed like a mother to me.'

Janet's story had a happy ending, and the way in which she wrote so fully about her experiences demonstrates the sense of satisfaction and achievement which the birth and mothering of Daniel brought to her, and through her to her whole family.

Her account of the help she received from Pauline and the midwife is a cameo of the effective helper described by Caplan (1969) and Weiss (1976). Both define effective support as that which enables the stressed individual to accept the helper as an ally, and which assures him or her that the helper's skill, time and understanding are available for as long as they are needed.

The secret of success in being such a helper lies in the relationship which develops between the individual and the care-giver. This relationship can be seen in a study of mothers who had unintended home deliveries because of the industrial action in hospitals in 1973. Goldthorpe and Richardson (1974) found that the dominant influence on the mother's reaction to labour was the relationship which she had with *her* midwife (their emphasis). They considered that this was because the community midwife's orientation was mother-centred, in contrast to the hospital regime which was routine-centred. It must also be pointed out, though, that the community midwives were highly delighted to have such an opportunity to display their competence at home deliveries, and this would have increased their commitment. The same pattern is seen in Shields' (1978) study of the satisfaction of women with their care during labour and delivery, in which the mothers rated the nurses' sensitivity and personal commitment to their needs more highly than their professional skills.

Both of these studies focus upon the support of women during labour and delivery, and the dearth of studies on post-natal care indicates the need for its concepts and organisation to be critically evaluated in order to develop consistently skilled, sensitive and integrated care.

The aims of post-natal care

The purpose of all maternity care is to enable a woman to be successful in becoming a mother, and this success applies not only to the physiological processes involved but also to the psychological and emotional processes which motivate the desire for parenthood and its fulfilment.

Birth, like death, cannot be avoided. Successful pregnancy leads inevitably to labour and birth, and to the joys and responsibilities of parenthood. However much parenthood is sought and welcomed, its irrevocable process brings tremendous physical and psychological change within a comparatively short period of time and this makes great demands upon a woman's emotional and psychological resources. The birth of the baby marks the watershed of those changes, and it is during this time that mothers are most in need of caring and sensitive support from their families and friends, and when the attitudes and caring skills of midwives and doctors have the most impact.

Childbirth and mothering should be a time of fulfilment and joy for both mothers and fathers, and the quality of the care which surrounds them should be a matter of concern for the whole of our society.

The latter half of the twentieth century has seen dramatic changes in the provision of skilled care for women during pregnancy, labour and childbirth. The establishment of the Health Service, the development of obstetric and paediatric knowledge and technology, and the improvement in the general health of the population have all served to reduce the levels of maternal and perinatal mortality to a degree undreamt of by the early pioneers of maternity care.

One of the most fundamental changes has been that the usual place for birth to take place is no longer the home, but the hospital. This marks a major change in the cultural patterns of childbirth in the West (Oakley 1977), and in the physical and psychological environment in which mothers and babies begin their lives together. The family to which they both belong is fragmented during this critical phase in their lives, with the mother and baby in hospital and the father, siblings and grandparents at home.

A good deal of attention has been drawn to the dangers of 'medicalising' childbirth, and many authors have argued that the desire to provide for the physical safety of mothers and their offspring has obscured, and at times ignored, their emotional and psychological needs (Riley 1977; Oakley 1977; Chard and Richards 1977; Kitzinger and Davis 1978; Chalmers 1978; Cartwright 1979, Great Britain 1980). As a result of this debate, there has been considerable relaxation and change in attitudes towards the care of women during labour, and in the way that parents and siblings are welcomed into special care nurseries (Romney and White 1984).

But little attention has been paid to the period after birth when the mother, her husband and their baby learn to care for one another, and during which time the pattern of their relationship with each other is established to a large degree. An unhappy woman will not be able to enter fully into this life-enhancing situation; she will feel that she is failing both her husband and her baby. Her self-image will be impairee, family relationships will be strained, and an experience which should be joyful and fulfilling may instead become one of frustration and disappointment.

The objectives of post-natal care are threefold and inter-related. They are: promoting the physical recovery of the mother and baby from the effects of pregnancy, labour and delivery; establishing sound infant feeding practices and fostering good maternal–child relationships; and providing the psychological support required to strengthen the mother's confidence in her-self, and in her ability to care for her baby, whatever her particu-lar personal, family or social situation may be.

The role of all who care for mothers, fathers and infants during the first days and weeks following childbirth should be centred upon nurturing the mother in such a way that she is able to adjust to the major changes which the baby has brought into her life, to become confident in caring for him, and to enjoy her developing relationship with him (Curry 1982). From this firm emotional base she will then be able to respond to the needs of her husband and family, and relationships will be strengthened enabling all the members of the family to give and receive the loving support which each one needs from the others.

Failings of the present system of post-natal care

The main focus of post-natal care has traditionally been that of ensuring the physical recovery of the mother from the effects of pregnancy and labour, and establishing infant feeding pat-terns. The emotional and psychological needs of mothers have not received much attention until recently, and there has been an assumption that these needs will automatically be met if the first two aspects of care are satisfied. The organisation of post-natal care has accordingly been based upon this premise.

Before the recommendations of the Peel Committee (Great Britain 1970) began to encourage delivery in hospital for all women, it was customary for those delivered in hospital to stay there for ten days after the birth. Women who were delivered in their own home received care from their community midwife for the same period of time. The increasing numbers of hospital deliveries led to a need for post-natal care to be shared between the hospital and community midwifery services, which were then administered by two separate authorities. As a result certain policies and agreements were made, upon which the transfer of mothers from hospital to community post-natal care was based.

The most common policy adopted was for the mother to be transferred to the care of the community midwife on the third day after the birth of her baby, and 61.9% of the mothers in this study went home on the third day. This, no doubt, was an administratively convenient time in which to make the necessary arrangements, but it ignored the fact that many women would prefer to go home, and be fit enough to go home, within a few hours of their baby's birth, while others would prefer for a variety of reasons to stay in the hospital for longer than 48 hours.

The adoption of 48 hours or 'three days' as the time when most mothers are transferred home means that the population of a post-natal ward is constantly changing, and this makes it very difficult for a relationship of trust and acceptance to develop between the mother and the midwife.

Another anomaly is the concept of the 'third' day after the birth. Somewhere in the mists of midwifery administration it was decided that if a baby was born before noon, that day was considered to be his 'first' day. However if he was foolish enough to be born one minute or more after noon, his 'first' day would not be recognised until the following day! Many women fail to see the point of this system: they expect to go home 48 hours after the birth and are disappointed when they are required to stay a further 24 hours in order to fulfil the criterion of discharge on the 'third' day.

This pattern of transferring the majority of mothers and babies home on the 'third' day was the major cause of the routine and chronological system of care which was observed in the post-natal wards. Mothers were expected to take responsibility for the care and feeding of their babies from the first or second day so that they could go home on the third day with some experience of meeting their baby's needs. Those mothers who were not able to cope with this system were then seen as 'having problems', and the whole pattern of care stifled the efforts of the midwives to give care and advice on an individual basis. The midwives frequently expressed their frustration at this rapid change-over of mother and babies, complaining that it was impossible for them to get to know any mother well unless she stayed in the ward for more than 48 hours.

Midwives and doctors working in the community have the opportunity to develop a continuing relationship with their clients. The primary care team consisting of general practitioner, midwife and health visitor can adopt a team approach to maternity care: they care for a comparatively small group of pregnant women at a time, and their relationship with the mother and her family continues after the baby has been born. Midwives and doctors working in hospital face a different situation. They do not have the advantage of meeting women in their own homes, but usually meet them for the first time in the somewhat impersonal setting of an ante-natal clinic. They provide care for women who face major problems in pregnancy and parturition, as well as those who can expect a normal labour and delivery, and they deal with large numbers of different women every year.

A considerable proportion of hospital staff are student and junior staff midwives, and medical students and junior medical staff. These staff members are younger, and less mature in life-skills than their colleagues in the primary care team, who will have had considerable experience in their respective professions before they become eligible to be part of such a team.

A further difficulty is created by the frequent movement of hospital staff. Student and staff midwives rotate around the various departments of a maternity hospital, and from day duty to night duty. Many student midwives do not continue as staff midwives once they have qualified, and of those who do practise as staff midwives, many leave after a short time either to pursue a different career in nursing or to embark upon motherhood themselves. Medical students also move around frequently, and junior medical staff may change their appointments every six months. These frequent changes make it difficult for junior medical and midwifery staff to develop consistent relationships with clients, or to develop inter-personal skills and confidence in caring for mothers. This situation encourages the continuation of routine approaches to care because such patterns help inexperienced staff to cope with the demands which are made upon them.

Another difficulty is that the development of hospital-based maternity care has been modelled upon the disease/diagnosis/treatment concepts of care which prevail in the acute sectors of the hospital service. As a result we tend to describe mothers by a form of hospital shorthand. We talk about women 'being delivered' rather than 'giving birth', and the mode of delivery becomes a code whereby we classify the 'diagnosis'. Thus we talk about a 'primip breech' or a 'normal delivery, gravida two', and this leads to an unconscious assumption about the care which such a mother will need.

The end result of all this has been to obscure the variety of client needs, and to stifle the development of woman-centred systems of care. This is particularly true of post-natal care, which tends to be given a lower status than the other aspects of maternity care.

The present study was undertaken in order to identify ways in which the psychological care of women could become an integral part of post-natal care. The final chapter of this book will be devoted to suggesting ways in which these results could be applied in order to provide the kind of care which will strengthen the confidence of mothers and enrich their experience of mothering. Such care is unlikely to be more expensive than the present system, but it will be more effective in achieving the objectives of post-natal care.

8

Developing a flexible support system

Caplan (1964) asserts that members of all the caring professions need to develop their knowledge and technical insight in order to practise the kind of work with their clients which will help them towards mental health as well as accomplishing the basic goals of the profession. He goes on to say that many professional care-givers are already achieving this quality of work with their clients on the basis of their own personality and life-experience, and this is certainly true of those who choose to work in the maternity services.

In order to fulfil Caplan's vision for all the women for whom the maternity services care, the kind of supportive environment needs to be created which is not an optional extra available to some women because of their special needs or because of the particular motivation and skill of individual doctors or mid-wives, but one which is an integral part of the organisational framework of the service.

Creating a flexible supportive environment has three key elements: recognising the uniqueness of each woman and enabling her to be free to be herself and not conform to any pre-judged or expected pattern of mothering; establishing a relationship of mutual trust and respect; and ensuring that all the different people involved in providing care work together in a consistent and co-ordinated manner.

The midwife has a key role to play in this situation. She is the member of the maternity services team who has most continuity of contact with a woman during the time of pregnancy, labour and the post-natal period, and she is the only member of the team whose work is solely concerned with the care of pregnant and parturient women.

Pregnancy, childbirth and the puerperium are a continuum and the care of mothers should be planned as a continuous process. There are, however, certain key stages in the process. These are: establishing relationships and planning the pattern of care during the ante-natal period, the climax of labour and birth and the first contact between the newborn and his or her parents, the time spent in the post-natal ward, and the beginning of a new family pattern when the mother and baby first return home.

The ante-natal period: developing a care plan

The foundations of effective care are laid during the woman's pregnancy by the establishment of a relationship through which her needs and desires can be discussed and certain options for care can be explored. Some women will have very clear ideas about the care they wish to receive in labour; others may choose to leave certain decisions in the hands of their midwife or doctor. The same applies to the pattern of post-natal care and decisions about the period of time the woman wishes to spend in hospital after the birth, and the factors which influence that decision.

The emphasis in these discussions should be upon the woman's right to exercise a choice, rather than on offering her pre-determined options. This will boost the self-confidence of those women whose opinions are rarely sought either by family or by figures in authority.

The resulting information must then be used in the planning of care, and it must be co-ordinated in such a way that it is available not only to all who become involved with caring for the woman as time goes on, but is identified as the basis upon which any other decisions about her care are made.

This process is initiated during the ante-natal period. The most usual way for it to begin is via the community midwife. A woman's first contact with the maternity services is normally when she sees her general practitioner to confirm pregnancy. This is usually followed by a visit made to the woman's home by the community midwife, and this visit is invaluable. The woman is on her own territory, and she and the midwife have an opportunity to talk freely together without the likelihood of interruption or the pressures of time which are to be found in ante-natal clinics. In this confidential situation the midwife can learn a good deal about the mother's personal and family circumstances that will influence the planning of the maternity care needed.

This visit can then become the basis of an individual maternity care plan, which can be updated as necessary and which in turn becomes the basis of care in the hospital as well as in the community.

The value of this approach was highlighted in the results of the study. The community midwives made three visits during the ante-natal period to the homes of all mothers booked for delivery in hospital 1. Their report was then used as a basis for the planning of co-ordinated care by the hospital and community services. The overwhelming majority of these mothers said that they felt they had a great deal of choice in the length of time they spent in the post-natal ward, and they scored significantly higher levels of satisfaction with their post-natal care in hospital than the mothers who were delivered in hospitals 2 and 3.

Building relationships in the busy setting of hospital ante-natal clinics is not as easy as in the community but has been achieved by creating small teams of midwives working in the hospital who care for a particular group of women.

Such teams can either care for all the women who are booked with a particular consultant (Hooton 1984; Cooper 1984), or take full responsibility for a group of low-risk women who are booked for a delivery in hospital under the care of the midwives (Flint 1985). These teams of midwives maintain contact with a woman all through pregnancy, and one or more members of the team will be available to care for her throughout labour, delivery and her stay in the post-natal ward. In some cases the post-natal care is continued in the woman's home by the midwife who cared for her in the hospital.

By a combination of these systems it is possible to collate and co-ordinate information about the woman's individual needs and preferences. Decisions which have been made about the conduct of labour can then be readily available to the midwife or doctor who is responsible for the mother's care at that time, even if she and the mother have never met before (Henschel 1982).

On the basis of discussions held with the mother, tentative plans can be made about the pattern of post-natal care, the length of time the woman wishes to spend in hospital and the arrangements which will need to be made by her family and the community midwife. It should be recognised, however, that plans made at this stage may need to be revised in the light of the events of pregnancy, labour and delivery, the mother's feelings once her baby is born, and any changes which may occur in the family circumstances. The mother may decide to go home earlier than she had planned or to stay in hospital longer. In all these things the final decision should be the mother's; it does not build up a woman's confidence in herself, or in her ability as a mother, to have her decisions brushed to one side by others.

For these reasons it is no longer appropriate for doctors or midwives working in hospital ante-natal clinics to fix a set time for women to stay in hospital – for example, to say that all primigravidae must stay in hospital for seven days – nor for community midwives to have to give their 'consent' before a woman can come home to their care. These are relics of the inter-authority agreements of the past and are no longer justified in a co-ordinated service. Neither is it appropriate for doctors on the post-natal wards to make arbitrary decisions which ignore previously agreed plans about when a woman may go home. The term 'may go home' is in any case an anachronism because there is no law which can compel a woman to stay in hospital.

The following comments received from one of the mothers in the study illustrate the distress which can result from this assumption that there is a pre-ordained 'correct' time for discharge from hospital:

> I was quite prepared to spend seven days in hospital until the doctor who saw me on the fourth day told me I would be able to go home the day after, only to have my hopes dashed by another doctor who saw me the day after, and said I couldn't go home that day. There was no change in my condition so the decision was just a personal opinion. I think doctors should have more consideration for their patients and no mention should be made about going home until they are absolutely certain. I spent two days in tears because of this doctor's thoughtlessness.

In addition to developing a co-ordinated care plan upon which midwives and doctors base total patient care, there is a need to consider the organisation and management of post-natal care. Post-natal care begins in the delivery suite, as soon as the birth is complete.

The 'fourth stage' of labour: enhancing satisfaction with motherhood

The results of the study showed that maternal satisfaction with motherhood acted as a boost to emotional well-being, and that it was enhanced by close contact between the mother and her baby during the first hour after delivery. For many of the women in the study this close contact was made possible because they breast fed their baby whilst they were still in the labour ward.

Most midwifery and obstetric text-books recognise three stages of labour: the first stage of dilatation of the cervix, leading to the second expulsive stage which results in the birth of the baby, followed by the third stage of expulsion of the placenta and contraction of the uterus to control haemorrhage. It is high time that a fourth stage of labour was recognised and became as important a part of the conduct of labour as the first three. This fourth stage is the time immediately following the birth when the mother and her newborn baby can come into close physical and emotional contact with each other. Although the work of Leboyer (1975), Klaus and Kennell (1982) and many others has stressed the importance of this contact, it still tends to be regarded as an optional extra which may be possible if circumstances are favourable.

Birth is preceded by forty weeks of pregnancy during which time the maternity services have taken great care to ensure the birth of a healthy baby to a healthy mother. It is perhaps indicative of the foreshortened view of midwives and doctors that birth is seen as the climax of care, and that although sharing the moment of birth with the parents is enjoyed, the bustle of clearing up after a delivery, writing up the records and arranging a post-natal bed tends to distract from the importance of enabling the parents and baby to spend an uninterrupted time together for as long as they wish.

The birth of their child is a peak experience in the life of its parents; it is a deeply emotional and personal moment which cannot be recaptured. When it is over the parents will separate for a time, the mother and baby going to the post-natal ward, and the father going home to spread the news to the rest of the family. Those who care for women during labour and childbirth should ensure that this period of time is regarded as sacrosanct and that nothing apart from immediate danger to the life of the mother or baby is allowed to disturb it. It is particularly important for the father of the baby, and his needs tend to be forgotten. He may not have an opportunity to be in such close contact with his infant for several days, and he may be going home exhausted but hopefully exhilarated by the experience he has just shared.

If the father of the baby is not with the mother during or immediately after the birth, she still needs to enjoy sharing this moment with some other companion or with the midwife or doctor who has cared for her during labour. The important thing is that she should be able to delight in her baby and to share that delight with someone else. She should also be praised for her achievement in giving birth; nothing saps joy or self-confidence more than an attitude which conveys that having a baby is a common occurrence and not particularly special!

The satisfactory completion of this stage of labour should therefore be regarded as requiring the same degree of attention and care as the first three stages, and no doctor or midwife should consider that his or her responsibilities are at an end until it has been fulfilled.

This fourth stage of labour will still need to be fulfilled even when it is not possible immediately after the birth either because the mother is anaesthetised or because the baby requires urgent attention or is stillborn. In the first instance a time of sharing between the baby's parents can be arranged as soon as the mother is able to enter into it fully, and the same pattern of uninterrupted time should be followed. If the baby is ill, the mother must be enabled to see and touch him before he is whisked away to special care. She and her partner may then need a time to comfort each other. When a stillbirth occurs, many parents find it helpful to see and touch the baby, delighting and grieving in his unfulfilled beauty and potential. This opportunity for parents to grieve together over a dead or sick baby is just as important as the time spent rejoicing over a healthy child, and nothing should be allowed to interfere with it.

Midwives have a particular role to play in ensuring that this fourth stage is fulfilled for all parents. Midwives are the key people in determining the way that delivery suites are run. It is the midwives who take responsibility for the conduct of the majority of births in this country, and where the labour does not result in a normal delivery, it is the midwife who takes over the care of the mother from the doctor and who organises the tranfer to the post-natal ward. Midwives therefore have a particular responsibility to ensure that the fostering of healthy parent–child relationships becomes an integral part of the care given, and that junior medical staff and medical and midwifery students are instructed in its significance.

The post-natal ward

After the peak experience of birth, the mother needs time to rest and recover from the physical stress of labour and delivery before she embarks upon the process of coping with all the demands which motherhood brings.

For the majority of women this process will begin in the post-natal ward of a hospital. Many women will prefer to go home as soon as possible after delivery, because they have had a normal labour and delivery and feel confident that they have the kind of help and support at home which will enable them to cope. Others will need to stay longer in order to recover from a difficult pregnancy, labour or delivery, or because the baby is in need of special care. Yet others will prefer to stay longer because they need time to become confident in feeding and caring for their baby, or because they lack help at home.

The results of the present study showed that two groups of women were particularly vulnerable to emotional distress: those with high trait anxiety levels, and those with a low self-image in feeding. Anxious women found it difficult to relax and feel at home in the ward, but lacked confidence when they went home. Those with low self-image in feeding were discouraged by conflicting advice and by comparing themselves with the 'mothering Jones's' in the next bed.

The care of these women poses a dilemma which can only be resolved by creating the kind of environment in the post-natal ward which will help the anxious woman to relax and will build

up the confidence of those with low self-esteem. This atmosphere will not only benefit all the mothers in the ward, but will
encourage staff to develop concepts of care which are woman-
centred rather than routine-centred.

There are two main ways of achieving such an environment:
changing the way in which post-natal wards are run and the
work organised, and enabling midwives to plan and carry out
a programme of co-ordinated and consistent care designed to
meet the individual needs of mothers.

Ward organisation

For a variety of reasons post-natal wards tend to be run on the
same pattern of organisation found in acute medical or surgical
wards. The pace of life on a post-natal ward is very fast because
so many mothers spend a very short period of time in it. As a
result a system has evolved where there are set times for carrying
out certain tasks so that they are not overlooked, which in turn
leads to midwives' 'rounds' in which the same task is carried
out for all mothers – the temperature round, medicine rounds
and a round to check the feeding charts of all the babies in the
ward. During the day the house officers also do rounds to see
either all the mothers or all the babies in the ward. They may
be followed by a phlebotomist or a physiotherapist, all with
their set quota of mothers to see. The domestic staff too have
their routine of work to follow, and meals arrive on the ward
at pre-determined times irrespective of the needs of mothers or
their babies.

All these activities produce a task- or routine-centred pattern
of care in which the mother as an individual is swamped and
her care is fragmented. This mould needs to be broken and the
ward run to suit the mothers.

First the 'diagnosis'-centred approach needs to be broken
down. The names of the mother and her baby should appear
at the top of any records or care plans and used whenever her
care is discussed, so that she is known as Mrs Mary Johnson
and Robert, rather than Mrs Johnson, gravida 2, normal delivery,
third day! The ward should be regarded as the mothers' territory
and the names of mothers and their babies should also be put
on the doors of four- or six-bedded bays or single rooms in
order to reinforce the woman's right to privacy.

Next, the pattern of the ward 'day' should be made to revolve around the mothers who are resident in it. The demands of a new baby make the prospect of a full night's sleep very unlikely, and this is particularly true of mothers who are breast feeding. Indeed recent research (Glasier *et al.* 1984) suggests that night-time suckling releases more prolaction than day-time suckling, thereby increasing lactation. The results of the present study, however, showed that lack of sleep caused considerable stress for all the mothers and was associated with low self-image in feeding. Mothers therefore need to be able to fit their sleeping patterns to those of their babies and to be able to rest and sleep at various intervals throughout the 24 hours. The current routine patterns of the day in a post-natal ward frustrate this need, so the pattern must be changed. The mother's need for rest must be considered a priority.

Many wards arrange a period in the day when the ward is closed, curtains are drawn and mothers are encouraged to rest. This pattern can be extended. Mothers should be supplied with 'Do not disturb' notices and all staff should be considered to be negligent in their care if they disturb a sleeping woman without good reason.

This is particularly important in the morning and there should be no scheduled time for starting the ward activity. Mothers who have had a disturbed night often fall into a deep sleep in the early hours of the morning. It is ridiculous to wake these women with a cup of tea at 6 or 7 a.m. followed by breakfast at 7.30 a.m. Instead mothers should be encouraged to sleep as long as they are able, and have a buffet-style breakfast when they are ready. The use of dishwashers will overcome any problems this creates for domestic work routines. Once the mothers are up and about, the activities of the ward day can begin.

Single rooms or, if these are not available, a particular part of a larger ward should be earmarked for the use of mothers who need to sleep during the day either because they have spent several hours in labour or because they had a disturbed night because of a restless baby. These rooms should be clearly marked 'Do not disturb' and no one, neither doctors, cleaners nor any other members of staff or visitors, should be allowed to disturb the mother until she has recovered.

These changes in the pattern of ward organisation will have

the effect of shifting the emphasis of the ward from that of a task- or routine-completion framework to one which varies from day to day according to the needs of the mothers in the ward. This in turn will mean that staff will no longer be valued for 'getting all the work done' but for being flexible in their approaches to care, and will encourage the further development of a relaxed environment which adapts itself to the needs of mothers rather than one in which the mothers are expected to fit into the existing hospital regime. One mother noted how much the pattern of post-natal care had changed since her first baby was born:

> My experience in hospital contrasted strongly with that of eight years ago when I had my first baby. At that time I had extreme difficulty in persevering with breast feeding as my baby did not conveniently fit her feeding pattern into the hospital timetable. This time the whole of my time in hospital was so enjoyable that I was in no rush to get home and cope on my own! The entire nursing staff were extremely helpful at a time when one naturally feels most insecure. One was allowed to do as much or as little as one wished with the baby, building up confidence gradually. Again this differed drastically from my earlier experience when there was a set programme of tasks for each day in hospital.

It is surprising how quickly midwives have been able to adapt their patterns and concepts of care once the existing regime has been questioned or the environment changed. This has been true of traditional patterns of care in labour (Romney and Gordon 1981) and in the rapid development of birthing rooms in maternity hospitals (Romney and White 1984).

Another situation arose recently in a maternity hospital which created a change in attitude and understanding. A double bed was installed in a single room on a post-natal ward. The room was attractively furnished and decorated and was made available for the use of couples who had suffered a stillbirth or whose baby was ill in the special care baby unit. This innovation had caused a few eyebrows to be raised and some sensational reporting in the local press! A number of the midwifery staff had felt a little uncomfortable at the prospect of having a husband sleeping in the ward at night.

One of the first to use the room were a couple whose baby was seriously ill in the special care unit, and whose prognosis was poor. On the second night after the baby's birth the husband awoke at 3 a.m. to find his wife in tears. She said that she knew their son was dying and that he might die before she had held him in her arms. The husband immediately went up to the special care baby unit where the infant's condition was very poor. He was invited to bring his wife in a wheelchair to the unit, where together they sat and cuddled their infant until he died a few hours later.

This incident changed the attitudes of the staff towards the double room. The midwives said that if the husband had not been there with his wife, they would have left her to sleep, believing that they were thus protecting her from the distress of knowing that her child was dying. Instead they saw that the parents and child needed to help each other through the experience of death and they felt privileged to share that experience with them (S.W.K. Skelton, personal communication). It is not easy to enter into the deep emotions of others but this is one of the reasons why midwives choose to follow their particular profession.

Caring for mothers and babies

Failings of the present system

Midwives gain deep satisfaction from being able to use their skills within a one-to-one relationship with a particular mother and her family, which is why so many enjoy working in the community. Frustration of this professional role is one of the reasons why midwives do not stay in their chosen career (Ashton 1982). This frustration was particularly prevalent among the midwives working in the post-natal wards, who complained that they were unable to build any kind of relationship with their clients or to give the kind of care which they believed mothers needed and which they desired to give. The main factors working against the provision of individualised care were the patterns of ward organisation and the routine-centred approach to care. These led to a lack of continuity of care and the problem of conflicting advice.

This was particularly true of the routine and chronological way in which mothers were expected to take increasing responsibility for the care and feeding of their babies. The same pattern was followed for all mothers irrespective of their age, previous experience with babies or physical state.

Apart from those mothers who had experienced a difficult birth or whose babies had been delivered by caesarian section, all were expected to take responsibility for the toilet needs of their baby within a few hours of the birth. This care was usually supervised by a nursery nurse, nursing auxiliary or student midwife who was allocated this responsibility for all mothers in the ward.

Breast feeding mothers received a good deal of help for the first few days after delivery, and this help was usually given by midwives. Bottle feeding mothers did not receive as much help, and although they were often shown how to give the first feed, very little supervision was given afterwards.

The mother's physical recovery and the involution of her uterus were checked daily by a midwife, and although there was some attempt to co-ordinate this aspect of care it was frequently carried out by different midwives on different days.

This pattern of work led to there being very little opportunity for the mothers to form any kind of consistent relationship with a particular midwife or other member of staff with whom they could discuss their particular needs. The routine approach also encouraged mothers to compare their prowess in caring for their babies with the expectations of midwives or other staff or with their neighbours in the rest of the ward, and this was very damaging to those mothers who needed a longer time to develop their confidence and skill because of their high degree of anxiety or their inexperience.

Conflicting advice made the situation worse, and had a marked effect upon the mother's self-image in relation to feeding her baby.

Self-image in feeding

When a woman is feeding her baby she is not just giving him food, but communicating her love and protection. She is rewarded and encouraged when the baby receives the food eagerly and benefits from her efforts. It is therefore extremely important for the mother to be confident that her baby is receiving the care that he needs, and that she is the key person who is able to fulfil those needs. This confidence takes some time to develop, and will depend upon the care and encouragement the mother receives. The over-riding principle in helping mothers to gain this confidence is that of encouragement and praise. If all goes well the mother becomes more confident and better still at looking after her baby, but nothing interferes more with the growth of empathy between a mother and her baby than failure (McKeith 1966).

The breast feeding mothers had an advantage in this process. They received a good deal of help and encouragement from midwives, although they also suffered from conflicting advice. But successful breast feeding reinforces the mother's role as the key person, indeed the only person, who can fulfil her baby's needs. The bottle feeding mothers on the other hand did not receive as much attention and therefore were not given as much encouragement and praise for their skill in providing for their babies' needs. This may be the reason why their self-image was much lower than that of the breast feeding mothers.

The lowest self-image was recorded by the mothers, both breast and bottle feeding, who became distressed about the feeding of their babies, and several of the breast feeders among them later gave up and bottle fed their babies. One of the dangers in the difficulty which may be present in the early days of breast feeding is that a member of staff or a member of the family may 'take over' and bottle feed the baby, thereby reducing the mother's role as the key person in fulfiling her baby's needs, and reinforcing her feeling of failure.

Mothers who are anxious about the feeding of their babies seek advice from numerous people. If this advice, especially from midwives or other professional staff, is conflicting then the mother becomes confused, and may conclude that the fault is hers and that she has failed in her key role towards her baby.

The effect of growing success or failure in this key role is seen in the mothers' scores on the Broussard-type scale. Mothers who said that their baby was doing 'better than average' had a high self-image in feeding in the early days in hospital and did not complain as much of conflicting advice, but a growing lack of confidence and possible disappointment in the baby's response is seen in the scores of those mothers whose self-image was low and who felt that their baby's progress at six weeks old was 'worse than average'.

Helping mothers to become confident, and identifying those who need to take things slowly and steadily, can only be achieved in a programme and pattern of care which will focus upon individual mothers and allow them the freedom to be different. It must be as frustrating for confident mothers who have successfully cared for their older children to have detailed supervision from a young and comparatively inexperienced midwife, as it is distressing for inexperienced mothers to be left to cope with little help. The present routine system of giving every woman the same pattern of care perpetuates this problem.

Planning care for individual mothers

The problem can, however, be overcome by a further change in the organisation of post-natal care which enables individual midwives to take the reponsibility for co-ordinating the care of individual mothers. This programme must be based upon the care plan formulated during the ante-natal period, and in which the tentative plans for post-natal care agreed between the mother and her community or team midwife have been recorded.

The process begins as soon as the post-natal ward staff are informed that a mother is coming to them from the delivery suite. Before the mother arrives the midwife should have read the details in her care plan and arranged for her to go into a single room or quiet area of the ward designated as the 'Do Not Disturb' area, so that she will be able to sleep after her efforts in labour. The midwife should then either go to the delivery suite to escort the mother and her baby to the post-natal ward, or be ready to greet her by name as she arrives in the ward. She will ensure too that mother and baby have spent some time together in the delivery suite and that the baby has been fed, before she settles the mother down for a rest.

While the mother is sleeping the midwife will have an opportunity to explore her history in full, so that once the mother is rested she can have a discussion with her. It is important to ensure privacy for this interview, and the midwife should sit at the side of the bed, at a lower level than the mother. As a result of this discussion certain plans are made and written into the care plan. The advice which is given about feeding, and any other arrangements which are made, should be written verbatim into the care plan so that other staff on the ward, and those who will care for the mother during other shifts, can follow the same pattern of advice.

The midwife who initiates this care plan will take the main responsibility for the care of the mother for the time she is in the ward. Other midwives will come into contact with the mother, but they will follow what has already been agreed and written in the care plan.

Conflicting advice can be further reduced by a daily staff discussion during which the needs of the mothers are discussed. This discussion should include all the ward team. Mothers often talk more to nursing auxiliaries and domestic staff because they tend to be older women with a motherly image. This tendency should be used for the benefit of the mothers, and nursing auxiliaries and domestics often have very revealing information to give: they may be aware of the mother who has put on a bright face to the midwife but has been weeping in the bathroom.

This pattern of work has been found to be effective in reducing the incidence of conflicting advice, changing the environment of a post-natal ward, and breaking down the routine patterns and building trusting relationships. It has resulted in increased satisfaction for mothers and for the midwives and other members of the ward team. Further details can be found in earlier work (Ball and Stanley 1984).

Going home from hospital

The length of time that a woman spends in hospital should be determined by her wishes, her confidence in caring for her baby, and by the kind of help she can expect to receive when she goes home.

The involution of the uterus and healing of the perineum take a number of weeks, and apart from those women who have been delivered by caesarian section, who have had a particularly difficult delivery, or suffering from a concurrent physical illness, physical status should not be the major criterion for discharge from hospital. However, because of the 'medical' model of hospital organisation the 'medical fitness' approach has tended to be used in determining the time for a woman to go home. This can play havoc if a junior house officer tells a mother she can go home when she and her midwife have agreed a process of gradually building up her confidence and skill in caring for herself and her baby.

It is high time this approach ceased, and arrangements for mothers to go home should be made by the midwife in charge of their care in the post-natal ward. It seems strange that a midwife, who is recognised by law and by hospital practice to be sufficiently skilled and competent to conduct labour and delivery, including taking responsibility for prescribing controlled drugs, topping up epidural analgesia, and intubating and resuscitating babies, is thought by the present system not capable of judging when a woman's post-natal physical condition would make her unfit to be discharged home. Also, the junior house officer has many other demands upon his time, and is not able as a result to have all the information which would enable him to make a balanced judgement of a mother's total needs.

These suggested changes in the organisation and patterns of post-natal care are not unique and many hospitals are developing them in order to provide a flexible and sensitive approach to the care of mothers and babies.

The steady growth of post-natal support groups, often run by health visitors or by mothers who have needed extra help themselves, are also a means of providing extra support and companionship.

Working together

At a recent conference concerned with the mental health of childbearing women it was suggested that as many as one woman in six suffers from some degree of emotional disturbance during the post-natal period, that approximately one in ten will develop post-natal depression and that this degree of incidence is found in all cultures (Cox 1985). The amount of personal and family distress related to these figures is considerable, and has serious implications for maternal and family welfare. Unless we accept this degree of distress as inevitable, surely it is not unreasonable to suggest that skilled and sensitive support might reduce the degree or prevent the development of post-natal emotional distress?

It is important to remember that post-natal distress and depression lie at one end of a whole spectrum of emotional reactions to motherhood, and that at the opposite end are those women who are very happy and content. The majority of women are somewhere in the middle, and would perhaps describe themselves as content and coping, even if not euphoric about motherhood. The pattern of emotional support for mothers, therefore, should be directed towards helping distressed mothers move along the spectrum towards the content and coping group, and the purpose of this book has been to assist those engaged in the care of mothers to identify those most at risk and to give them the kind of care they need.

Most studies of post-natal distress or depression emphasise those events and circumstances which had a detrimental effect upon emotional well-being at the expense of others which enhanced and enriched the mothering experience. The results and comments presented in this book have emphasised the effects of uncoordinated care and conflicting advice, but it would be erroneous to leave the impression that they are representative of all the comments made by mothers in the study. Many mothers wrote to express their appreciation of and satisfaction with the care they received from midwives, doctors and health visitors. Nevertheless, the study did identify problems in post-natal care which could be avoided, and the willingness to face and overcome such problems is the hallmark of any profession (Stewart 1982).

This book has concentrated upon the work of midwives rather than other members of the obstetric team, and I hope that the new insights which have been gained will earn me the forgiveness of obstetricians, paediatricians, general practitioners, health visitors, physiotherapists and all the other professions concerned with mothers and babies. Midwives do have a particular contribution to make, however, and their role has been somewhat overlooked if not ignored by previous studies of factors affecting transition to motherhood (Robinson, Golden and

Bradley 1980). The close contact which exists between mothers and midwives, especially during labour and the puerperium, gives midwives a unique opportunity to observe and to influence a woman's response to the demands which motherhood makes upon her.

But no single professional or consumer group has the monopoly of concern for the welfare of mothers and babies, nor does any group possess all the skills and attributes needed to help women from many different backgrounds and with varying degrees of maturity to realise their full potential as mothers. It is as part of a team, in which all members co-operate, and value the contribution made by the others, that the caring, supportive environment will be created which mothers have the right to expect.

It is important that all professionals concerned with the care of mothers and babies resist the tendency to be defensive about their respective roles and practices and stifle their eagerness to apportion blame for problems which arise. Instead they need to develop a willingness to listen and learn from each other and from their clients, and to recognise that facing and overcoming problems and criticism is the hallmark not only of any profession, but particularly of those who seek to maintain the highest standards of service and integrity.

References

Allport, G.W. (1961). *Pattern and Growth in Personality*. Holt, New York.

Arnold, M. (1960). *Emotion and Personality*. Columbia University Press, New York.

Ashton, R.M. (1982). Where do we go from here? *Midwives Chronicle*, **95** (1131), 119–21.

Bacon, C.J. and Wylie, J.M. (1976). Mothers' attitudes in infant feeding at Newcastle General Hospital in 1975. *British Medical journal*, **i**, 308–9.

Ball, J.A. (1981). The effects of the present patterns of maternity care upon the emotional needs of mothers: I, II and III. *Midwives Chronicle*, **95**, (1120), 150–4; (1121), 198–202; (1122), 231–3.

Ball, J.A. (1983ª). The effect of the present patterns of maternity care upon the emotional needs of mothers with particular reference to the post-natal period. MSc Thesis, Dept of Nursing, Manchester University.

Ball, J.A. (1983ᵇ). Moving forward in post-natal care: some aspects of a research project. (Supplement: RCM Professional Day Papers.) *Midwives Chronicle*, **96** (1149), 13–16.

Ball, J.A. (1984). What happens now? (RCM Supplement.) *Nursing Times*, **80** (29), 3–5.

Ball, J.A. and Stanley, J. (1984). Stress and the mother. (Supplement: RCM Professional Day Papers.) *Midwives Chronicle*, **97** (1162), xviii–xxii.

Beck, A.T., Ward, C.H., Mendelson, M., Mock, J. and Erbaugh, J. (1961). An inventory for measuring depression. *Archives of General Psychiatry*, **4**, 561–71.

Bernal, J. (1972). Crying during the first ten days of life and maternal response. *Developmental Medicine and Child Neurology*, **4**, 362–72.

Bowlby, J. (1951). *Maternal Care and Mental Health*. Bulletin of the World Health Organisation. HMSO, London.

Bowlby, J. (1961). Separation anxiety: a critical review of the literature. *Journal of Child Psychology*, **15**, 9–52.

Boyd, C. and Sellers, L. (1982). *The British Way of Birth*. Pan Books, London.

Brady, J.V., Porter, R.W., Conrad, D.G. and Mason, J.W. (1958). Avoidance behaviour and the development of gastro-duodenal ulcers. *Journal of the Experimental Analysis of Behaviour*, **1**, 69–72.

Bronfenbrenner, U. (1958). Socialization and social class through time and space. In *Readings in Social Psychology*, ed. E.E. Maccoby, T.M. Newcomb and E.L. Harley. Henry Holt, New York.

Broussard, E.R. and Hartner, M.S.S. (1971). Further considerations regarding maternal perception of the newborn. In *Exceptional Infant: Studies in Abnormality*, Vol. 2, ed. J. Jerome, pp. 432–49. Brunner-Mazel, New York.

Brown, G. and Harris, T. (1978). *Social Origins of Depression: A Study of Psychiatric Disorder in Women*. Tavistock Publications, London.

Brown, W.A. (1979). *Psychological Care during Pregnancy and the Post-natal Period.* Raven Press, New York.

Caplan, G. (1964). *Principles of Preventative Psychiatry.* Tavistock Publications, London.

Caplan, G. (1969). *An Approach to Community Mental Health.* Tavistock Publications, London.

Caplan, G. and Killilea M. (1976). *Support Systems and Mutual Help.* Grune and Stratton, Orlando, Florida.

Cartwright, A. (1979). *The Dignity of Labour?* Tavistock Publications, London.

Cattell, R.B. and Scheier, I.H. (1961). *Meaning and Measurement of Neuroticism and Anxiety.* Ronald Press, New York.

Chalmers, I. (1978). Implications of the current debate on obstetric practice. In *Place of Birth*, ed. S. Kitzinger and J Davis. Oxford University Press, London.

Chard, T. and Richards, M. (eds.) (1977). Lessons for the future. In *Benefits and Hazards of the New Obstetrics*, pp. 157–63. Heinemann, Medical Books, London.

Chertok, L. (1969). *Motherhood and Personality.* Tavistock Publications, London.

Clayton, S. (1979). *Maternity Care: Some Patients' Views.* Newcastle Community Health Council Survey Report. NCHC, Newcastle.

Cooper, I.G. (1984). Midwifery team allocation. (Supplement: RCM Professional Day Papers.) *Midwives Chronicle*, **97** (1161), vi–vii.

Cox, B.S. (1974). Rooming in. *Nursing Times*, **70**, 1246–7.

Cox, J. (1978). Some socio-cultural determinants of psychiatric morbidity associated with childbearing. In *Mental Illness in Pregnancy and the Puerperium*, ed. M. Sandler, pp. 91–8. Oxford University Press.

Cox, J. (1985). Paper given at a joint conference of the Marcé Society and Royal College of Midwives, Kings Fund Centre, London, 8 March 1985.

Curry, M.A. (1982). *Parent–Infant Bonding.* C.V. Mosby, St Louis.

Dalton, K. (1964). *The Pre-menstrual Syndrome.* Heinemann Medical Books, London.

Dalton, K. (1971). Prospective study into puerperal depression. *British Journal of Psychiatry*, **118**, 689–92.

Dalton, K. (1980). *Depression after Childbirth.* Oxford University Press.

Derlega, V.J. and Janda, L.H. (1978) *Personal Adjustment: The Psychology of Everyday Life.* General Learning Press (subsidiary of Scott, Foresman and Co.), Glenview, Illinois.

Dewi-Rees, W. and Lutkin, S.G. (1971). Parental depression before and after childbirth. *Journal of the Royal College of General Practitioners*, **21**, 26–31.

Draramraj, C., Siac, G., Kierney, C.M., Harper, R.C., Pareck, A. and Weissman, B. (1981). Observations on maternal preference for rooming-in Harper facilities. *Paediatrics*, **67**(5), 638–40.

Dunn, J.B. and Richard, M.P.H. (1977). Observation of the developing relationship between the mother and baby in the neonatal period. In *Studies in Mother–Infant Interaction*, ed. H.R. Schaffer, pp. 427–53. Academic Press, London.

Dyer, E.D. (1976). Parenthood as crisis: a re-study. In *Human Adaptation: Coping with Life Stress*, ed, R.H. Mous, pp. 177–85. D.C. Heath and Co., Lexington, Mass.

Erikson, E.H. (1959). Identity and the life cycle. *Psychological Issues*, **1**, 1–165.

Erikson, E.H. (1963). *Childhood and Society*, 2nd edn. Norton, New York.

Eysenck, H.J. (1959). *Manual of the Maudesley Personality Inventory.* University of London Press.

Eysenck, H.J. and Eysenck, S.B.G. (1968). *Manual of the Eysenck Personality Questionnaire*. Hodder and Stoughton Educational Division, Kent.

Eysenck, H.J., Soueif, M.I. and White, P.O. (1969), A joint factoral study of Guildford, Cattell and Eysenck scales. In *Personality Structure and Measurement*, ed. H.J. Eysenck and S.B.G. Eysenck, pp. 171–93. Routledge and Kegan Paul, London.

Ferreira, A.J. (1960). The pregnant mother's emotional attitude and its reflection upon the newborn. *American Journal of Orthopsychiatry*, 30, 553–61.

Filshie, S., Williams, J., Osbourn, M., Senior, O.E., Symonds, E.M. and Backett, E.M. (1981). Post-natal care in hospital: time for a change. *International Journal of Nursing Studies*, 18(2), 89–95.

Flint, C. (1985). Labour of Love. *Nursing Times*, 81(5), 16–18.

Franklin, B.L. (1974). *Patient Anxiety on Admission to Hospital*. Royal College of Nursing, London.

Freud, S. (1940). *The Outline of Psychoanalysis*. Hogarth Press, London.

Freud, S. (1957). *Civilisation and its Discontents*, transl. J. Riviere (1st edn 1930). Hogarth Press, London.

Frommer, E.A. and O'Shea, G. (1973). Antenatal identification of women liable to have problems in managing their infants. *British Journal of Psychiatry*, 123, 149–56.

Glasier, A.D., McNeilly, A.S. and Howie, P.W. (1984). Free prolactin response to suckling. *Clinical Endocrinology*, 10, 109–16.

Goldberg, D.P., Cooper, B., Eastwood, M.R., Kedward, H.B. and Shepherd, M. (1974). A standardized psychiatric interview for use in community surveys. *British Journal of Preventative and Social Medicine*, 24, 18–23.

Goldthorpe, W.C. and Richardson, J. (1974). Reorganisation of the Health Service: a comment on domiciliary confinement in view of the hospital strike 1973. *Midwife, Health Visitor and Community Nurse*, 10, 265–70.

Great Britain: Department of Health and Social Security (1970). *Domiciliary Midwifery and Maternity Bed Needs*. Report of the Sub-Committee, Central Health Services Council, Standing Maternity and Midwifery Advisory Committee. HMSO, London.

Great Britain: Department of Health and Social Security (1980). *Perinatal and Neonatal Mortality*. Second Report from the Parliamentary Social Services Committee 1979–1980, HMSO, London.

Great Britain (1982). *Birth Statistics*. Review of the Registrar General Birth and Family Building in England and Wales. HMSO, London.

Gruis, M. (1977). Beyond maternity: post-partum concerns of mothers. *American Journal of Maternal–Child Nursing*, 2(3), 182–8.

Hales, D.J., Lozoff, B., Sosa, R. and Kennell, J.H. (1977). Defining the limits of the maternal sensitive period. *Developmental Medicine and Child Neurology*, 19, 454.

Hayward, J. (1975). *Information: A Prescription Against Pain*. Royal College of Nursing, London.

Henschel, D. (1982). Comments in *Parent–Infant Bonding*, by M.H. Klaus and J.H. Kennell, pp. 99–109. C.V. Mosby, St Louis.

Hilgard, E.R., Atkinson, R.L. and Atkinson, R.C. (1979). *Introduction to Psychology*, 7th edn. Harcourt, Brace Jovanovich, New York.

Holmes, T.H. and Rahe, R.H. (1967). Social readjustment rating scale. *Journal of Psychosomatic Research*, 11, 219.

Hooton, P. (1984). The team approach to midwifery care. (Supplement: RCM Professional Day Papers.) *Midwives Chronicle*, 97,(1161), v–vii.

Houston, M.J. (1981). Breast feeding: success or failure. *Journal of Advanced Nursing*, **6**, 447–54.

Hytten, F.E., Yorkston, J.M. and Thomson, A.M. (1958). Difficulties encountered with breast feeding. *British Medical Journal*, **I**, 310–15.

Jackson, E.D., Wilke, L.C. and Auerbeck, H. (1956). Statistical report on incidence and duration of breast feeding in relation to personal, social and hospital maternity factors. *Paediatrics*, **17**, 700–12.

Janis, I.L. (1958). *Psychological Stress: Psychosomatic and Behavioural Studies of Surgical Patients*. Wiley, New York.

Kennell, J.H., Chesler, D., Wolfe, H., Jerauld, R., McAlpine, W., Kreger, N.C., Steffa, M., and Klaus, M.H. (1974). Maternal behaviour one year after early and extended post-partum contact. *Developmental Medicine and Child Neurology*, **16**, 172–9.

Kennell, J.H., Trause, M.A. and Klaus, M.H. (1975). Evidence for a sensitive period in the human mother. In *Parent–Infant Interaction*, ed. E. Porter and M. O'Connor, pp. 87–101. Ciba Foundation Symposium No. 33. Associated Scientific Publishers, Amsterdam.

Kitzinger, S. (1978). *Women as Mothers*. Martin Robertson, Oxford.

Kitzinger, S. and Davis, J. (eds.) (1978). *Place of Birth*. Oxford University Press, London.

Klaus, M.H. and Kennell, J.H. (1970). Human maternal behaviour at first contact with her young. *Pediatrics*, **46**(2), 187–92.

Klaus, M.H. and Kennell, J.H. (1976). *Maternal–Infant Bonding*. C.V. Mosby, St Louis.

Klaus, M.H. and Kennell, J.H. (1982). *Parent–Infant Bonding*. C.V. Mosby, St Louis.

Klaus, M.H., Jerauld, R., Kreger, N.C., McAlpine, W., Steffa, M. and Kennell, J.H. (1972). Maternal attachment: importance of the first post-partum days. *New England Journal of Medicine*, **286**, 460–3.

Klaus, M.H., Trause, M.A. and Kennell, J.H. (1975). Does human maternal behaviour after delivery show a characteristic pattern? In *Parent–Infant Interaction*, ed. E. Porter and M. O'Connor, pp. 69–85. Ciba Foundation Symposium No. 33. Associated Scientific Publishers, Amsterdam.

Kumar, R. and Robson, K. (1978). Neurotic disturbance during pregnancy and the puerperium. In *Mental Illness in Pregnancy and the Puerperium*, ed. M. Sandler, pp. 40–51. Oxford University Press.

Laryea, M. (1984). *Post-Natal Care: The Midwife's Role*. Churchill Livingstone, London.

Lazarus, R.S. (1966). *Psychological Stress and the Coping Process*. McGraw-Hill, New York.

Lazarus, R.S. (1969). *Patterns of Adjustment and Human Effectiveness*. McGraw-Hill, New York.

Leboyer, F. (1975). Birth Without Violence. Wildwood House, London.

Leiderman, P.H. and Seashore, M.J. (1975). Mother–infant separation: some delayed consequences. In *Parent–Infant Interaction*, ed. E. Porter and M. O'Connor, pp. 213–39. Ciba Foundation Symposium No. 33. Associated Scientific Publishers, Amsterdam.

Lishman, A. (1972). Selective factors in memory. II. Affective disorders. *Psychological Medicine*, **2**, 248–53.

Llewellyn Davies, M. (1979). *Maternity: Letters from Working Women*. Virago Press, London.

Lynch, M.A., Roberts, J. and Gordon, M. (1976). Child abuse: early warning in the maternity hospital. *Development Medicine and Child Neurology,* **18,** 759–66.

McKeith, R. (1966). How can we help the mother to adapt to her child? *Proceedings of the Royal Society of Medicine,* **59,** 1013–18.

Maslow, A.H. (1970). *Motivation and Personality.* Harper and Row, New York and London.

Mechanic, D. (1962). *Students under Stress.* Free Press, New York.

Mintz, A. (1951). Non-adaptive group behaviour. *Journal of Abnormal and Social Psychology,* **46,** 150–9.

Mischel, W. (1968). *Personality and Assessment.* Wiley, New York.

Newton, N. (1955). *Maternal Emotions.* Harper and Row., New York.

Nilsson, A. (1972). Parental emotional adjustment. In *Psychosomatic Medicine in Obstetrics and Gynaecology,* ed. N. Morris. Wiley, New York.

Nuckalls, C.B., Cassell, J. and Kaplan, B.H. (1972). Psycho-social assets, life-crises and the prognosis of pregnancy. *American Journal of Epidemiology,* **95,** 431–4.

Oakley, A. (1977). Cross-cultural practices. In *Benefits and Hazards of the New Obstetrics,* ed. T. Chard and M. Richards. pp. 18–33. Heinemann Medical Books, London.

Oakley, A. (1980). *Women Confined.* Martin Robertson, Oxford.

Oppenheim, A.N. (1966). *Questionnaire Design and Attitude Measurement.* Heinemann, London.

Perkins, E. (1979). Ante-natal care and post-natal nursing. In *Health Education in Practice,* ed. D.C. Anderson, pp. 105–23. Croom Helm, London.

Pitt, B. (1968). 'Atypical' depression following childbirth. *British Journal of Psychiatry,* **114,** 1325–35.

Pitt, B. (1978). Introduction. In *Mental Illness in Pregnancy and the Puerperium,* ed. M. Sandler, pp. 1–6. Oxford University Press.

Reiff, R. (1966). Cited in Lazarus, R.S. (1969). *Patterns of Adjustment and Human Effectiveness,* pp. 327–9. McGraw-Hill, New York.

Riley, E.D.M. (1977). What do women want? The question of choice in the conduct of labour. In *Benefits and Hazards of the New Obstetrics,* ed. T. Chard and M. Richards, pp. 62–71. Heinemann Medical Books, London.

Robinson, S., Golden, J. and Bradley, S. (1980). The midwife: a developing or diminishing role? In *Post-Natal Care: The Midwife's Role.* Churchill Livingstone, Edinburgh.

Romney, M. and Gordon, H. (1981). Is your enema really necessary? *British Medical Journal,* **283,** 1269–72.

Romney, M.L. and White, U.G.L. (1984). Current Practices in Labour. In *Perinatal Nursing,* ed. P.A. Field, pp. 63–80. Churchill Livingstone, Edinburgh.

Rosen, B. and Stein, M.J. (1980). Children and abusive women. *American Journal of Diseases of Childhood,* **134,** 946–51.

Seligman, M.E.P. (1975). *Helplessness: On Depression, Development and Death.* W.H. Freeman, San Francisco.

Shannon, I.L. and Isbell, G.M. (1963). Stress in dental patients. Technical Report No. SAM-TDR-63-29, USAF School of Aerospace Medicine. Cited in *Lazarus (1969).*

Shields, D. (1978). Nursing care in labour and patient satisfaction. *Journal of Advances in Nursing,* **3**(6), 535–50.

Siegel, S. (1956). *Non-parametric Statistics for the Behavioural Sciences*, International Student Edition. McGraw-Hill, New York.

Stewart, A. (1982). What are our opportunities? The personal and professional development of the midwife. *Midwives Chronicle*, **95**(1130), 84–6.

Stopher, P.R. and Meyburg, A.H. (1979). *Survey Sampling and Multivariate Analysis for Social Scientists and Engineers*. Lexington Books (D.G. Heath and Co.), Lexington, Mass.

Stott, D.H. (1962). Evidence for a congenital factor in maladjustment and delinquency. *American Journal of Psychiatry*, **118**, 781–94.

Stott, D.H. (1973). Follow up study from birth of the effects of pre-natal stresses. *Developmental Medicine and Child Neurology*, **15**, 770–87.

Theobald, G.W. (1959). Home on the second day: the Bradford experiment. *British Medical Journal*, **ii**, 1364–7.

Tod, E.D.M. (1964), Puerperal depression: a prospective epidemiology study. Lancet, **II**, 1264.

Topliss, E.P. (1970). Selection procedures for hospital and domiciliary confinements. In *In the Beginning*, ed. G. McLachlan and R. Shegog, pp. 59–78. Oxford University Press.

Totman, R. (1979). *Social Causes of Illness*. Souvenir Press, London.

Weinmann, J. (1981). *An Outline of Psychology as Applied to Medicine*. John Wright, Bristol.

Weiss, R.S. (1976). Transition states and other stressful situations: their nature and programs for their management. In *Support Systems and Mutual Help*, ed. G. Caplan and M. Killelia. pp. 211–32. Grune and Stratton, New York.

Wilson-Barnett, J. (1979). *Stress in Hospital: Patients' Psychological Reactions to Illness and Health Care*. Churchill Livingstone, Edinburgh.

Wilson-Barnett, J. and Carrigy, A. (1978). Factors influencing patients' emotional reaction to hospitalization. *Journal of Advanced Nursing*, **3**(3), 221–9.

Wolkind, S. (1981). Depression in the mothers of young children. *Archives of Diseases of Children*, **56**, 1–3.